LIVING LONG
LIVING WELL

A Comprehensive Guide to Living a Healthier, Happier and longer life

By

Richard C. Jimison

TABLE OF CONTENTS

INTRODUCTION

The Transformative Journey of Living Long and Well

In the center of a city, where time moves quickly and the pulse of life beats relentlessly, there once lived a man whose story exemplified the repercussions of ignoring the fragile vessel we call our bodies. His name, long forgotten by many, resonated down the corridors of anonymity until the day our paths crossed.

Meet John, a man who, like so many of us, has danced through life without paying attention to his aging body's whispers. With each passing day, John was sprinting towards premature aging by indulging in culinary delights without hesitation, embracing sedentary habits, and ignoring sleep as a mere inconvenience.

One fateful day, our paths crossed, and I met the man desperate to escape the chains of his own carelessness. Little did John know that the answer to living a better, happier, and longer life was within grasp.

In the following pages, I will tell the story of John's remarkable transformation—a metamorphosis that defied the usual narrative of irreversible decline. John not only slowed but reversed the aging process by following meticulously prepared health-enhancing advice. His restoration was nothing short of miraculous, and the world saw a man reborn, shedding years like a snake does its old skin.

What happened in John's life is a source of hope and inspiration for everybody who finds themselves at the crossroads of neglect and rediscovery. This book, Living Long, Living Well: A Comprehensive Guide to Living a Healthier, Happier, and Longer Life, is more than just a collection of wisdom; it demonstrates the transformational ability that each of us possesses.

As you continue on your trip through the pages that follow, keep in mind that the information contained inside these chapters has the power to transform your life, just as it did for John. It is my earnest opinion that with the thoughts and techniques outlined in this book, you, too, may create a road to a future full of vitality, joy, and the gift of many more years.

Welcome to a life well lived.

CHAPTER 1

Understanding the Secrets of Longevity

The Longevity Diet Explained

Throughout history, humanity has sought longevity, or the desire to live a longer and healthy life. In recent years, the concept of a "Longevity Diet" has received a lot of attention.

This nutritional approach is more than just losing a few pounds; it is a comprehensive lifestyle designed to promote total well-being and improve quality of life. We will look at the Longevity Diet's philosophy, science, and practical applications.

Nutrient-Rich Foods

The Longevity Diet focuses on nutrient-dense meals. This entails selecting foods with a high concentration of vitamins, minerals, antioxidants, and other vital nutrients per calorie.

The emphasis is not solely on calorie restriction, but also on maximizing the nutritional value of each meal. Think of it as quality vs. quantity.

Fruits, vegetables, whole grains, nuts, and seeds are featured prominently. These foods are high in antioxidants, which help the body resist oxidative stress, a major contributor to aging and age-related disorders.

The Longevity Diet promotes a colorful plate, as different colors in fruits and vegetables often represent distinct nutrient profiles.

Mindful Eating

Beyond the sorts of food, the Longevity Diet focuses on how we consume foods. Mindful eating is an essential component of this technique. In a fast-paced world where meals are sometimes rushed, taking the time to savor and appreciate each bite can have a significant impact on digestion and overall happiness.

Mindful eating entails staying present during meals, paying attention to hunger and fullness indicators, and enjoying the sensory experience of eating. Individuals who have a positive relationship with food can create a long-term and balanced approach to nutrition.

Intermittent Fasting

The Longevity Diet is renowned for its use of intermittent fasting. This technique entails alternately eating and fasting, resulting in periods of no food consumption. Intermittent fasting has been related to improved metabolic health, cellular repair mechanisms, and potentially increased longevity.

Popular strategies include the 16/8 method (16 hours of fasting followed by an 8-hour eating window) and the 5:2 approach (eating regularly for five days and ingesting relatively few calories on two non-consecutive days). Intermittent fasting is consistent with the body's natural circadian rhythm and may improve autophagy, a process that eliminates damaged cells while regenerating new, healthy ones.

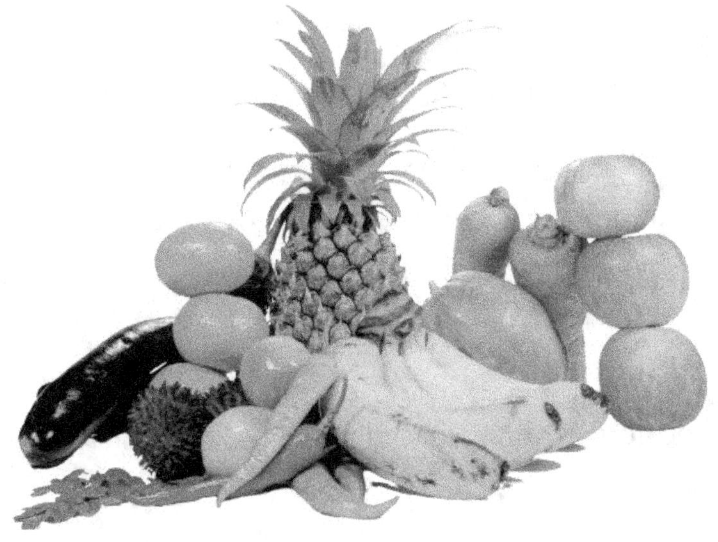

Healthy Fats

Contrary to previous fat-phobic movements, the Longevity Diet promotes healthy fats, notably omega-3 fatty acids. Omega-3 fatty acids are well-known for their anti-inflammatory effects and function in brain health.

A balanced diet of omega-3 and omega-6 fatty acids is essential, as an imbalance can lead to inflammation. The Longevity Diet recommends including these healthy fats into your meals to improve cardiovascular health and cognitive performance.

Plant-Based Focus

While not entirely vegetarian or vegan, the Longevity Diet promotes a plant-based approach to protein consumption. Legumes, beans, tofu, and tempeh are great protein sources, providing a variety of important amino acids without the health risks associated with heavy meat eating.

This trend toward plant-based proteins is consistent with research indicating that plant-rich diets may lead to a longer and healthier life. The Longevity Diet recognizes the role of protein in muscle growth and overall body function, while emphasizing choices that are sustainable and ethical.

Hydration and Longevity

Despite the emphasis on solid foods, the Longevity Diet recognizes the necessity of hydration. Adequate water intake is necessary for several biological activities, including digestion, vitamin absorption, and detoxification. Hydration promotes healthy skin, joints, and organs, resulting in a general sense of well-being.

The Longevity Diet promotes water as the primary beverage, while herbal teas are frequently used for their antioxidant benefits. Limiting sugary drinks and caffeine intake is recommended because they can upset the body's natural equilibrium and potentially contribute to inflammation.

Social Interaction and Eating Habits

The Longevity Diet recognizes the social aspect of eating. Cultivating a sense of community via shared meals has been linked to increased mental health and longevity. The emphasis on sharing meals with others, practicing appreciation, and cultivating positive social ties all contribute to a more holistic approach to well-being.

One of the most important foundations in the quest for a longer, better life is food. When we examine the complex relationship between nutrition and lifespan, the adage "you are what you eat" takes on new meaning.

Understanding the basics

A longevity diet does not revolve around deprivation or severe eating habits. Instead, it is about making intelligent, long-term decisions that nourish and support the body's natural functions. A well-balanced and diverse diet rich in vitamins, minerals, antioxidants, and other bioactive components serves as the foundation. Instead of focusing solely on calorie counting, the emphasis is on the quality of calories taken.

The Role of Fruits and Vegetables

Fruits and vegetables play a key role in plant-powered longevity. A large body of studies has demonstrated the benefits of a plant-based diet for longevity. Fruits and vegetables are high in antioxidants, fiber, and phytochemicals, which help to fight inflammation and oxidative stress, two factors that contribute to many age-related disorders.

The variety of hues found in fruits and vegetables represents a wide range of nutrients, each with its own significance in fostering cellular health.

Whole grains and legumes provide energy and vitality

Whole grains and legumes are the foundation of a diet that provides energy and promotes vitality. Rich in complex carbs, fiber, and important nutrients, these meals give a consistent release of energy, avoiding the spikes and crashes associated with refined carbohydrates.

Furthermore, they improve intestinal health and satiety, which aids in weight management—an important element in lifespan.

Moderation and Mindful Eating

Aside from specific food choices, the way we eat plays an important role in a longevity diet. Mindful eating, which includes paying attention to hunger and fullness cues, developing a connection with the sensory components of eating, and savoring each bite, has been linked to healthier food choices and better digestion. Furthermore, adopting moderation in portion sizes helps to maintain weight and reduces the risk of obesity-related disorders.

Intermittent fasting is a dietary strategy for longevity. Intermittent fasting, an eating pattern that alternates between periods of eating and fasting, has gained popularity due to its possible longevity advantages. According to research, intermittent fasting may increase cellular repair processes, promote autophagy (the body's mechanism for cleaning away damaged cells), and improve metabolic health.

However, it is critical to approach intermittent fasting in a balanced manner and consult with healthcare professionals, particularly for people with certain health conditions.

Nutrient-Rich Diet

One of the most important aspects of living a longer and healthier life is the fuel we give our bodies—nutrition. For millennia, the complicated dance between the foods we eat and our general health has piqued people's interest and investigation. As we investigate the role of nutrition in longevity, we discover the enormous effect that a nutrient-dense diet may have on not just our bodies but also our lifetime.

A nutrient-rich diet is really about giving our bodies with the necessary building blocks to function properly. It goes beyond the simplistic perspective of food as a source of energy and delves into the numerous vitamins, minerals, antioxidants, and other bioactive components that are essential for human health.

The body cannot create essential nutrients on its own, thus they must be obtained through diet. These include vitamins A, C, D, E, and K, minerals like calcium, magnesium, and potassium, as well as phytochemicals found in fruits, vegetables, and whole grains.

Antioxidants

Antioxidants, or substances that resist oxidative stress in the body, are important to the concept of a nutrient-rich diet. Oxidative stress occurs when there is an imbalance between the body's generation of free radicals and its ability to neutralize them. Free radicals, which are unstable chemicals created during numerous metabolic processes, can cause cell damage and contribute to aging and age-related disorders.

Fruits and vegetables, particularly those in brilliant hues, are high in antioxidants. Berries, leafy greens, and citrus fruits contain a variety of these defensive chemicals. By including a variety of colorful foods into our diets, we provide our bodies with the tools they require to combat the ravages of time.

Macronutrients and Micronutrients

A nutrient-dense diet acknowledges the relevance of macronutrients and micronutrients in sustaining health and enhancing longevity.

Carbohydrates, proteins, and lipids are all macronutrients, with each serving a specific purpose. Carbohydrates supply energy, proteins help with muscle function and repair, while fats are required for fat-soluble vitamin absorption and cell membrane maintenance.

Micronutrients include vitamins and minerals, which are needed in lower amounts but are equally important. These micronutrients serve as cofactors in a variety of physiological processes, affecting anything from bone health to immunological function.

The idea is to achieve a balance that meets the demands of each individual. While popular diets frequently emphasize specific macronutrient ratios, a nutrient-rich diet promotes a diverse and inclusive approach, ensuring that the body receives a wide range of vital nutrients.

Gut Health

Emerging study illuminates the complex relationship between our nutrition, intestinal health, and longevity. The gut microbiome, a complex ecology of billions of microorganisms in our digestive tract, is essential for nutritional absorption, immunological function, and even mental wellness.

A fiber-rich diet, including fruits, vegetables, and whole grains, promotes a healthy microbial community. These fibers work as prebiotics, supporting healthy bacteria in the gut. In turn, these bacteria create short-chain fatty acids, which have been related to better gut health and overall well-being.

Fermented foods such as yogurt, kefir, and sauerkraut offer probiotics—live beneficial bacteria—that help maintain a healthy gut microbiota. The complex relationship between diet and gut health highlights the necessity of seeing nutrition as a whole, integrated system.

The Mediterranean Paradigm

The Mediterranean diet is an excellent example of a nutrient-dense diet that has been shown to promote longevity. This dietary pattern, which includes an abundance of fruits and vegetables, whole grains, olive oil, and lean proteins, has been linked to a lower risk of heart disease, diabetes, and certain malignancies.

The Mediterranean diet is high in omega-3 fatty acids from fish, monounsaturated fats from olive oil, and a variety of antioxidants from colorful vegetables, demonstrating the synergistic advantages of a broad and nutrient-dense diet. It not only nourishes the body but also satisfies the palate, demonstrating that longevity can be a flavorful and delightful experience.

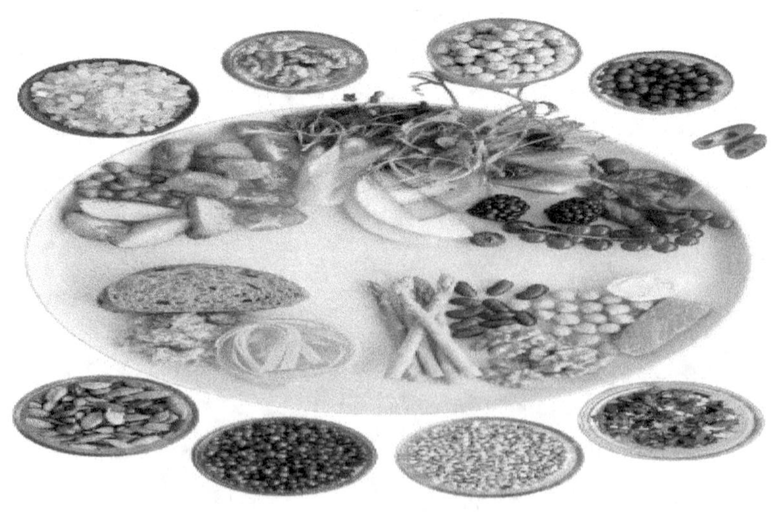

Personalization

While there are general rules for a nutrient-rich diet, it is critical to recognize the diversity of nutritional requirements. Age, gender, exercise level, and underlying health issues all have an impact on dietary requirements. A life-sustaining diet is a dynamic and customized journey rather than a one-size-fits-all prescription.

Adopting a nutrient-dense diet necessitates self-awareness and a grasp of how various foods affect personal well-being. Consulting with healthcare specialists or registered dietitians can give personalized counsel, ensuring that nutritional choices are in line with specific health objectives and needs.

Longevity beyond the Plate

A nutrient-dense diet is essential for longevity, but it is only one piece of the jigsaw. The combination of lifestyle factors such as adequate sleep, regular physical activity, stress management, and social relationships has a greater impact on overall well-being and longevity.

The Longevity Diet is not about strict restrictions or deprivation, but rather about developing a healthy and sustainable relationship with food. It celebrates the pleasure of eating, the social aspects of sharing meals, and the satisfaction of nourishing the body with foods that promote vitality.

Creating a Balanced and Sustainable Diet

In the world of nutrition, the concept of a balanced and sustainable diet stands above passing trends and crash diets. It's a strategy that not only feeds the body but also promotes long-term health. We will learn the concepts, advantages, and practical suggestions for creating a balanced and sustainable diet, building the groundwork for a happier life.

A healthy diet revolves around balance. It entails integrating a wide range of meals to ensure that the body receives a balanced supply of critical nutrients. This is more than just a single meal or a day's intake; it refers to the general makeup of one's diet over time.

The first step toward balance is to carefully incorporate macronutrients (carbohydrates, proteins, and fats). Carbohydrates supply energy, proteins help muscles operate and repair, and lipids are necessary for many biological functions, including hormone generation and nutrition absorption.

Balance diet also applies to micronutrients, which are vitamins and minerals that play important roles in a variety of physiological processes. A diet high in fruits, vegetables, whole grains, and lean proteins provides an adequate quantity of these micronutrients.

Diversifying dietary sources is the key to achieving equilibrium. Different foods provide different nutrients, and combining a rainbow of fruits and vegetables, whole grains, nuts, seeds, and lean meats results in a nutritional symphony that benefits the body in a variety of ways.

The Power of Portion Control

In a society where super-sized portions and unlimited buffets are the norm, portion control has emerged as a critical component of developing a balanced diet. It is not about deprivation, but rather about recognizing the body's requirements and giving it with the appropriate amount of nourishment.

Using the plate approach is a straightforward way to apply portion control. Divide your dish into three sections: half for veggies, one quarter for lean protein, and one quarter for whole grain. This visual guide ensures that the food is balanced and properly portioned.

Quality over Quantity

Building a balanced diet is much more than just fulfilling caloric requirements; it is also about getting the most nutritious value out of every calorie taken. Nutrient density is a guiding principle that emphasizes the necessity of eating foods high in vitamins, minerals, and other healthy substances.

Vibrant fruits and vegetables are high in nutrient richness. Their vibrant colors indicate the presence of a variety of antioxidants and phytochemicals that provide numerous health advantages. Including a variety of colors on your plate promotes a nutritious dinner.

Whole grains, lean proteins, and healthy fats are key components of a nutrient-dense diet. Choosing whole, unadulterated foods over refined versions ensures a higher concentration of important nutrients while avoiding unneeded additives.

Sustainable Eating

The quest for a balanced diet is intertwined with the broader concept of sustainability—a diet that not only promotes human health but also contributes to the health of the world. Sustainable eating entails making choices that reduce environmental impact while promoting long-term food security.

Choosing locally produced and seasonal produce helps to lessen the carbon footprint of food transportation. It also benefits local farmers by providing fresher, more flavorful ingredients.

While plant-based diets are gaining popularity due to their sustainability, not everyone may want to completely forgo meat. In such instances, conscious meat consumption is critical. Choosing lean, sustainably sourced meats and plant-based proteins helps to create a balance between nutritional requirements and environmental effect.

A sustainable diet includes not only what we eat, but also what we leave out. Minimizing food waste through good storage, meal planning, and creative use of leftovers is consistent with the ideals of sustainability.

The Role of Hydration in Balance

Hydration is sometimes overlooked in favor of solid foods, despite the fact that it is an essential component of a well-balanced diet. Water is required for digestion, nutritional absorption, temperature regulation, and the proper operation of all cells in the body.

Daily Hydration Goals: The "eight glasses a day" rule is a straightforward guideline, although individual hydration requirements can differ depending on age, activity level, and climate. Paying attention to thirst cues and drinking water consistently throughout the day maintains proper hydration.

Beyond Water: While water is the primary hydrating beverage, herbal teas and infusions can help to supplement total fluid consumption. Limiting sugary drinks and caffeine consumption promotes a healthy balance and reduces needless caloric intake.

Flexibility is an indicator of a healthy and balanced diet. When developing a nutritional plan, it is important to consider individual needs, preferences, and cultural concerns. A one-size-fits-all strategy frequently falls short, and the goal is to achieve a personalized balance that is appropriate for one's own circumstances.

Cultural Considerations: Traditional diets often reflect generations of nutritional understanding. Integrating ethnic dietary practices that stress complete, locally sourced foods can improve both nutritional and culinary outcomes.

Food Sensitivities and Allergies: For people who have unique dietary limitations or sensitivities, finding balance may require imaginative replacements and paying close attention to nutritional needs. Consulting with a healthcare expert or nutritionist can help you create a balanced diet that meets these requirements.

Sustainable Weight Management

A balanced and sustainable diet is not a quick fix for weight loss, but rather a comprehensive approach to general health. Crash diets and harsh limits can produce quick results, but they are frequently unsustainable in the long run. Sustainable weight control entails developing habits that maintain a healthy weight over time.

Slow and steady wins the race: Gradual, long-term reforms are more likely to be maintained than sudden, restrictive measures. Focusing on small, attainable goals and building on successes over time creates a solid basis for long-term change.

Physical exercise as a Companion: While nutrition is an important part of weight management, physical exercise complements it. Regular exercise not only aids in weight loss, but also improves general health and well-being.

CHAPTER 2

Exercise for Life

Few measures are more effective than regular physical activity for living a longer, healthier life. The benefits of exercise for life extend far beyond the constraints of a gym or scheduled training routine.

We will look at the many benefits of physical activity, including the science, practicalities, and various ways to incorporate movement into daily life for a life full of energy and well-being.

The Science of Exercise and Longevity

The link between exercise and longevity is strongly embedded in scientific knowledge. Numerous studies have repeatedly demonstrated the benefits of regular physical activity on general health and longevity. The body of data supports exercise's transforming potential, ranging from cardiovascular benefits to improved cognitive functioning.

Regular exercise strengthens the heart, increases blood circulation, and reduces blood pressure. These variables all contribute to a lower risk of cardiovascular disease, which is the leading cause of death worldwide.

Physical activity is essential for maintaining a healthy metabolism. Regular exercise regulates blood sugar levels, improves insulin sensitivity, and aids in weight management, lowering the risk of type 2 diabetes.

Exercise has a favorable impact on mental health in addition to its physical benefits. Regular physical activity has been linked to lower levels of anxiety and depression, increased mood, and better cognitive performance.

Chronic inflammation is a prevalent factor in many age-related illnesses. Exercise has been demonstrated to lower systemic inflammation, creating an environment conducive to lifespan.

Moving Beyond the Gym

While the gym remains an important place for regular training, the key of exercise for longevity is its incorporation into daily life. It's about developing a movement-focused lifestyle that goes beyond scheduled workout times. Here are practical methods to incorporate extra fitness into your daily routines:

Active Commuting: Walk or cycle instead of driving wherever possible. If your office is an acceptable distance away, consider incorporating these active ways of transportation into your daily routine.

Take the Stairs: While elevators can be handy, taking the stairs is a simple and effective approach to work your muscles and raise your heart rate. Over time, this minor shift might have a large impact on overall physical activity levels.

Lunchtime Walks: Take a quick walk during your lunch break. Whether it's around the workplace or in a neighboring park, this lunchtime exercise not only promotes physical activity but also refreshes the mind.

Desk workouts: To combat the sedentary aspect of office job, use desk workouts. Simple stretches, leg lifts, and seated marches can help break up extended periods of sitting.

Household chores can serve as a workout. Vacuuming, gardening, and cleaning can be surprisingly effective at raising your heart rate and engaging various muscle groups.

The Benefits of Strength Training in Longevity

While aerobic exercise is frequently the focus, strength training is an important component of a well-rounded fitness regimen. Building and maintaining muscle mass provides a range of benefits that are associated with longevity which includes:

Bone Health: Strength training helps to preserve bone density, lowering the incidence of osteoporosis and fractures, particularly as we age.

Metabolism Boost: Muscle tissue consumes more calories at rest than fat tissue. Strength training in your regimen boosts your metabolism, which contributes to weight management and overall metabolic health.

Functional Independence: Strong muscles promote functional independence by helping people to execute everyday tasks with ease and lowering the chance of falls and accidents.

Strength training has an impact on hormonal balance by boosting the release of growth hormone and testosterone. These hormones serve critical functions in sustaining vitality and countering the consequences of aging.

Mindful Movement Practices (Yoga and Tai Chi.)

Beyond traditional forms of exercise, mindful movement activities such as yoga and tai chi have gained popularity for their overall health benefits. These techniques effortlessly mix physical activity with mental well-being, providing a unique path to longevity:

Yoga: known for its emphasis on flexibility, balance, and breath control, is a low-impact workout that promotes joint health and mental clarity. Regular yoga practice has been linked to reduced stress, increased mood, and a higher overall quality of life.

Tai Chi: is a peaceful and flowing practice based on traditional Chinese martial arts, emphasizing slow, deliberate motions. It has been demonstrated to improve balance, prevent falls in older persons, and promote mental and emotional well-being.

Nature's Role in Physical Activity

Connecting with nature increases the advantages of physical activity. Outdoor activities not only provide a change of scenery, but they also mix movement with the restorative effects of nature.

Hiking: Exploring hiking paths not only works out different muscle areas, but it also helps people to connect with nature. The varied terrain adds a level of difficulty, improving cardiovascular fitness and overall well-being.

Riding: Whether on mountain routes or city paths, riding is a great outdoor sport. It mixes cardiovascular exercise with the thrill of discovery, resulting in a sustainable and fun approach to keep active.

Swimming: Natural bodies of water and outdoor swimming pools provide options for aquatic fitness. Swimming is a full-body workout that is easy on the joints and offers a refreshing alternative to traditional land-based hobbies.

Nature Walks & Bird Watching: A simple walk through a park or nature reserve can be a rejuvenating type of exercise. Bird watching instills curiosity, changing a walk into a conscious investigation of the natural world.

Mind-Body Connection (Meditation and Longevity)

The mind-body link is an important element of longevity, and meditation provides a unique opportunity to investigate this relationship. While not a typical kind of physical activity, meditation contributes to overall well-being and supplements more strenuous workouts.

Stress Reduction: Chronic stress is linked to aging and age-related illnesses. Meditation, which emphasizes awareness and relaxation, has been demonstrated to lower stress hormones and generate a sense of peace.

Cognitive Benefits: Meditation activities, such as mindfulness meditation, have been related to increased cognitive function, memory, and attention. These cognitive benefits help to keep the mind healthy and active throughout life.

Quality of Sleep: Adequate, peaceful sleep is essential for longevity. Meditation can improve sleep quality by calming the mind and increasing relaxation, benefiting both physical and mental health.

Community Engagement and Social Fitness

Exercise does not have to be something you do alone. The social dimension of physical activity is critical to maintaining long-term involvement and reaping the benefits of a socially active lifestyle:

Group courses: Participating in group exercise courses, whether in a gym or in the community, provides not just physical advantages but also a sense of companionship. Group activities may be both motivating and pleasant, turning fitness into a social event.

Team Sports: Participating in team sports promotes camaraderie, teamwork, and healthy competition. Team sports, such as soccer, basketball, and recreational leagues, provide a dynamic and exciting method to stay active.

Walking or Running Clubs: Starting or joining a walking or running club fosters a supportive network of like-minded people. The social aspect provides accountability and transforms exercise into a social event.

Dance Classes: Dance is a fun form of physical activity that incorporates movement and music. Taking dance classes, whether traditional or modern, not only gives a wonderful workout but also serves as a creative and social outlet.

A Personalized Path to Lifelong Wellbeing

Starting a journey toward sustainable health entails more than just working out; it also entails creating an exercise regimen that is tailored to individual interests, goals, and lifestyle.

Let's look at the concepts of personalizing a workout program for long-term well-being.

Understanding Your Personal Fitness Goals

Before putting on those sneakers, it's critical to establish personal fitness goals. Having specific goals, whether they are for weight control, cardiovascular health, strength growth, flexibility improvement, or a holistic well-being approach, serves as the foundation for a tailored exercise routine.

Weight Management: For people looking to manage or decrease weight, a combination of cardiovascular exercise, strength training, and mindful eating is required. The goal is to create a calorie deficit that can be sustained through increased activity and balanced nutrition.

Cardiovascular Health: Individuals looking to improve their cardiovascular health should prioritize aerobic activity. Brisk walking, jogging, cycling, swimming, and high-intensity interval training (HIIT) are all options for cardiovascular exercise.

Strength Building: Incorporating resistance training into your regimen is essential for increasing muscular growth and strength. Weightlifting, bodyweight exercises, and functional motions involving several muscular groups are all examples of this.

Flexibility Improvement: Flexibility is an important part of total fitness. Yoga, Pilates, and dynamic stretching practices can help improve flexibility, minimize the risk of injury, and increase mobility.

Holistic Well-Being: For people seeking a well-rounded approach to health, combining cardio, weight training, flexibility work, and contemplative activities such as yoga or meditation gives a holistic and long-term solution.

Striking a balance between cardiovascular and strength training

Achieving long-term health requires a combination of cardiovascular exercise and strength training. Each component provides distinct benefits that enhance overall well-being.

Cardiovascular exercise raises the heart rate, improves circulation, and increases respiratory function. Regular aerobic workouts help with weight control, improve mood through endorphin production, and promote cardiovascular health.

Strength training promotes lean muscle mass, which is essential for metabolic health, bone density, and functional independence. It also helps to prevent age-related muscle loss and promotes a healthy body composition.

Finding the Balance: Tailoring a workout plan entails striking the correct balance between cardiovascular and strength training based on personal goals and preferences. This could include alternating days, including both parts into each session, or focusing on key phases of a training cycle.

Implementing Functional Fitness

Functional fitness emphasizes activities that mirror real-life movements and increase general functionality. This method not only improves daily tasks, but it also helps to prevent injuries and maintain long-term health.

Bodyweight Exercises: Using bodyweight exercises such as squats, lunges, push-ups, and planks works numerous muscle groups while improving overall strength and stability.

Functional Movements: Exercises that mimic ordinary activities, such as bending, lifting, and reaching, help with functional fitness. These movements enhance balance, coordination, and mobility.

Stability Training: Using stability balls, resistance bands, or balance exercises can improve core strength and stability. A strong core is essential for general functional fitness.

Multidimensional Workouts: Incorporating exercises involving several joints and muscle groups enhances functional fitness over isolated motions. This may include kettle bell swings, medicine ball tosses, or TRX suspension training.

Sustainable health is a journey rather than a destination. Setting realistic and gradual goals ensures that the training regimen adapts to individual abilities and aspirations.

Breaking down long-term ambitions into manageable short-term goals gives you a sense of accomplishment and inspiration. These goals can be based on frequency, intensity, duration, or specific fitness achievements.

To encourage ongoing improvement, gradually raise the difficulty of workouts. This may include altering weights, increasing resistance, or advancing to more difficult routines.

Life is a dynamic process in which circumstances change. A sustained fitness routine responds to these changes. If time limits or other things disrupt the program, having alternate training options encourages consistency.

Prioritizing recovery and rest

Rest Days: Including rest days in your weekly routine helps your body recuperate and minimizes burnout. Rest allows the body to mend and strengthen itself, adding to overall resilience and sustainability.

Sleep Quality: Proper sleep is critical for recovery and general health. Adequate and restful sleep promotes hormone balance, muscle healing, and cognitive performance, all of which are necessary for long-term health.

Active Recovery: Incorporating low-intensity activities, such as walking or mild stretching, on rest days stimulates blood circulation and aids in recovery without putting too much strain on the body.

While creating an exercise regimen can be a personal activity, getting professional advice provides a layer of experience and assures that the activities chosen are appropriate for individual needs and health concerns.

Fitness Professionals: Certified fitness trainers, physical therapists, and exercise physiologists can offer tailored advice based on individual goals, fitness levels, and pre-existing health concerns.

Health Screenings: Before starting a new fitness routine, especially if you have pre-existing health concerns, you should speak with a healthcare practitioner. Health checks can aid in determining any potential hazards or limits.

Progress Check-ins: Reassessing fitness goals on a regular basis, reviewing progress, and changing the training regimen as needed to ensure that it remains in line with individual aspirations and capabilities.

CHAPTER 3

Cultivating a positive mindset for mental health and longevity.

The rich tapestry of lifespan reveals mental well-being as a thread sewn into the fabric of total health. The significant link between thought and lifespan is becoming more recognized, shedding light on the transforming effects that a positive attitude may have on our physical, emotional, and cognitive health.

I will uncover the subtle interplay between attitude, mental well-being, and longevity, traversing research, practical techniques, and the significant influence of our ideas on the path to a longer and happier life.

The Power of Positive Thinking

The concept of positive thinking is central to the relationship between mentality and longevity. This is not about mindless optimism, but rather a mindset that favors constructive, positive, and solution-oriented thinking.

Positive thinking has been shown to provide a wide range of advantages beyond mental health.

Stress Reduction: Positive thinking has been associated with lower levels of stress. When faced with a challenge, those with a positive mindset are more likely to address it with resilience and a problem-solving attitude, which reduces the detrimental effects of stress on the body.

Emotional Resilience: Developing a positive mentality helps to build emotional resilience—the ability to recover from setbacks and traverse life's ups and downs gracefully. This resilience is an important aspect in sustaining mental health throughout time.

Improved Coping Mechanisms: A positive attitude boosts coping mechanisms in the face of hardship. People who have a positive outlook are more likely to seek help, use effective problem-solving skills, and preserve a sense of autonomy in difficult situations.

The Mind-Body Connection's Impact on Physical Health

The mind and body are inextricably linked, and the impact of attitude goes beyond mental well-being to physical health. Emerging study investigates how positive thinking can improve longevity and general health.

Studies have found a link between pleasant emotions and cardiovascular health. People with a positive outlook may have lower blood pressure, a lower risk of heart disease, and better overall cardiovascular function.

Immune System Function: The immune system's reaction is affected by mental health. Positive emotions have been linked to a stronger immune system, which improves the body's ability to fight off diseases and illnesses.

Inflammation Reduction: Chronic inflammation contributes to a variety of age-related conditions. Positive thinking has been associated to decreased levels of inflammatory markers, indicating that it may have a role in reducing the risk of inflammatory disorders.

Neuroplasticity: Preparing the Brain for Longevity

The notion of neuroplasticity emphasizes the brain's extraordinary ability to adapt, rearrange, and generate new neural connections throughout time. Positive thinking has a significant impact on the structure and function of the brain, influencing cognitive health and increasing longevity.

Cognitive Resilience: A positive outlook has been linked to cognitive resilience—the ability to retain cognitive function while adapting to brain changes. This resilience plays a critical role in lowering the risk of cognitive decline and neurodegenerative disorders.

Enhanced Learning and Memory: Positive emotions have been linked to better learning and memory. The brain's plasticity allows for the creation of new neural pathways, which improve cognitive ability and mental agility.

Stress Mitigation: Chronic stress is harmful to the brain, weakening memory and cognitive function. Positive thinking and stress-reduction practices contribute to a healthy brain environment, which promotes cognitive lifespan.

Mindfulness and Longevity

Mindfulness, which has its roots in ancient contemplative practices, has risen to prominence in contemporary concerns about mental health. This present-centered method entails growing awareness of the present moment while accepting thoughts and feelings without judgment. Mindfulness practice has been linked to a variety of mental health and longevity advantages.

Mindfulness methods like meditation and mindful breathing are effective stress relievers. Individuals can interrupt the cycle of chronic stress and its negative consequences on mental and physical health by focusing their attention in the present.

Mindfulness improves emotional regulation by encouraging nonreactive observation of feelings. This enables people to respond to emotions in a controlled manner, minimizing impulsivity and improving emotional well-being.

Quality sleep is essential for lifespan, and mindfulness activities help to enhance sleep patterns. Mindful relaxation practices can help calm the mind and ease the transition into restful sleep.

Develop a Resilient Mindset

Cultivating a positive mindset and mental well-being entails making deliberate efforts to develop resilience—the ability to adapt to challenges and maintain equilibrium in the face of adversity. Resilience is a skill that may be learned and increased over time.

Adopting a Growth Mindset entails viewing problems as opportunities for learning and development. Individuals with a growth mentality see setbacks as transient and use them as stepping stones to progress.

Cultivating appreciation: Expressing appreciation is a simple yet effective approach to shift focus to the positive parts of life. Regularly identifying and appreciating what one is grateful for promotes a healthy mindset and adds to general well-being.

Fostering Social Connections: Social support is an essential component of resilience. Building and sustaining strong social connections gives a network of support during difficult times, which boosts mental health.

Developing Coping techniques: Identifying and implementing effective coping techniques is essential for resilience. This could include problem solving, seeking support, practicing self-compassion, or participating in activities that offer joy and fulfillment.

The Influence of Mindset on Lifestyle Decisions

Mindset has a direct impact on mental and physical health, as well as lifestyle choices that promote longevity. Individuals' mindsets often influence how they handle food, exercise, sleep, and stress management.

Healthy Lifestyle Choices: A happy mentality is linked to a greater possibility of adopting and keeping healthy lifestyle habits. This includes engaging in regular physical activity, eating nutritious foods, getting enough sleep, and properly managing stress.

Resilience in the Face of Setbacks: People with a positive outlook are more likely to recover from setbacks in their lifestyle choices. Instead than viewing a lapse as a failure, they see it as an opportunity to learn and improve their methods.

Consistent Well-Being Practices: One's mindset determines the consistency of their well-being practices. Those who take a positive attitude are more likely to adopt stress-relief activities, mindfulness techniques, and other healthy behaviors into their everyday life.

Promoting Mental Health across the Lifespan

Cultivating a healthy mindset and supporting mental health is a lifetime process. The ideas and behaviors that contribute to a happy attitude are useful at all phases of life, boosting resilience and increasing longevity.

Adolescence and Identity: Adolescence is a time of substantial identity formation. Developing a positive mindset during this phase entails cultivating self-compassion, increasing resilience, and supporting a growth mindset in the face of adversity.

Adulting and Life problems: Adulthood presents its own set of problems, including employment, relationships, and cultural expectations. A positive mindset becomes an invaluable advantage in overcoming these hurdles, encouraging adaptation and a sense of purpose.

Senior Years and Cognitive Health: As people get older, it becomes increasingly important to preserve their cognitive health. A positive outlook, paired with continual cognitive stimulation and social involvement, helps to build cognitive resilience in the senior years.

How to Develop a Resilient Mindset

In the uncertain journey of life, resilience serves as a beacon of strength—a quality that enables people to recover from failures, face adversity bravely, and negotiate challenges with grace.

Developing a resilient attitude entails not only weathering obstacles, but also seeing them as chances for growth and learning.

1. Adopting a growth mindset

At the heart of resilience is the concept of a growth mentality, which holds that abilities and intelligence can be enhanced through devotion and hard work. This mindset, created by psychologist Carol Dweck, views setbacks as opportunities for learning and growth rather than insurmountable barriers.

Shift from Fixed to Growth: Recognize and question fixed mindset beliefs, which hold that abilities are innate and immutable. Accept problems as opportunities to learn, persevere in the face of setbacks, and see effort as a means of achieving mastery.

Cultivate a Love of Learning: Encourage curiosity and a desire to learn new skills and knowledge. Approach problems with a desire to learn, realizing that each hurdle is a unique opportunity for personal and professional growth.

Celebrate work and Progress: Recognize and celebrate the work put in to overcome problems, regardless of the outcome. Recognizing the importance of perseverance reinforces the concept that resilience is a dynamic process of ongoing progress.

2. Practice Self-Compassion

Self-compassion is a great ally on the path to resilience, providing a calm and supportive perspective during challenging circumstances. It entails treating oneself with love, comprehending and acknowledging that imperfection is a common human experience.

Cultivate a Mindful Presence: Self-awareness is the foundation of mindfulness, which is essential for self-compassion. Mindfulness methods such as meditation or deep breathing can help you stay present and build a nonjudgmental awareness of your thoughts and emotions.

Challenge Self-Critical thinking: When confronted with misfortune, people frequently resort to self-critical thinking. Question these negative narratives by asking, "What would I say to a friend in this situation?" Extend the same kindness toward oneself as one would to a close friend.

Practice Self-care: Treat yourself with the same care and understanding that you would show a loved one. Instead of harsh self-criticism, use helpful and encouraging language to build resilience.

3. Developing Social Connections

Resilience is frequently fostered within the framework of social relationships. Strong relationships provide emotional support, offer alternative viewpoints, and form a network that strengthens an individual's ability to overcome obstacles.

Cultivate Supportive Relationships: Establish and maintain solid bonds with friends, family, and supportive people. Openly share your sentiments and concerns, as sharing experiences develops a sense of belonging and alleviates the load of hardship.

Join Community or Interest Groups: Participate in activities that match with your personal interests or passions. Participating in community or interest organizations allows you to connect with like-minded people, building a sense of community and shared purpose.

Seek Professional Support: Seeking professional help during a difficult time is a display of strength. Therapists, counselors, and support groups provide a secure environment for people to express their emotions, acquire insights, and receive help on how to build resilience.

4. Improving Problem-Solving Skills.

Resilience entails not only overcoming problems, but also actively participating in issue solving. Developing excellent problem-solving abilities allows people to tackle challenges with a sense of autonomy and resourcefulness.

Breaking down overwhelming tasks into smaller, attainable actions makes them more bearable. Identify particular components of the problem that can be addressed, and develop a plan for resolution.

Explore Different views: Resilient people approach problem resolution with a flexible mentality, taking into account multiple views and potential solutions. This versatility enables innovative problem-solving and increases the possibility of identifying effective alternatives.

Learn from Setbacks: Seeing setbacks as opportunities to learn is critical to developing resilience. Reflect on previous obstacles, identify lessons gained, and apply acquired knowledge to future problem-solving efforts.

5. Creating realistic goals and expectations

Individuals who set realistic goals and keep fair expectations experience increased resilience. Balancing ambition with an appreciation of one's limitations reduces stress and promotes a sense of success.

Break down Long-Term Goals: Ambitious, long-term goals might be scary. Break them down into smaller, more manageable benchmarks that provide a sense of accomplishment and success along the road. Celebrate each milestone to have a happy attitude.

Acknowledge Achievements: Celebrate all achievements, no matter how minor. Recognizing accomplishments maintains a good mindset and offers incentive to pursue larger goals.

6. Cultivating gratitude

Gratitude is a transforming approach that redirects the attention from life's obstacles to its positive features. Cultivating a grateful mentality improves resilience by instilling a sense of abundance and appreciation.

Keep a daily thankfulness notebook to focus on the positive aspects of your day. Recognizing moments of thankfulness, no matter how great or small, fosters a good outlook and combats negative thinking.

Express Gratitude to Others: Take the time to thank friends, family, and coworkers. Communicating appreciation not only enhances relationships, but it also promotes pleasant emotions, which boosts resilience.

Focus on the Present Moment: Gratitude frequently thrives in the present moment. Engage in mindfulness activities that focus on the present moment and encourage awareness of the good components in one's immediate environment.

7. Improving Emotional Regulation Skills

Resilience entails managing a wide range of emotions with ability and awareness. Developing emotional regulation abilities allows people to respond to situations with emotional intelligence, which promotes adaptability and well-being.

Identify and Label Emotions: Understanding and identifying emotions is the first step toward building resilience. Identify the precise feelings you're experiencing, as self-awareness is the foundation for good emotional management.

Mindful breathing is an effective method for emotional management. When confronted with strong emotions, take deliberate and deep breaths to calm the mind and create a pause for logical replies rather than impulsive ones.

Cultivate a Positive Emotional Toolkit: Create a set of skills for uplifting and managing emotions. This may include engaging in enjoyable activities, receiving support from others, or using creative outlets to express and process feelings.

8. Seeking Meaning and Purpose.

A resilient attitude is strongly linked to a sense of meaning and purpose in life. Finding purpose serves as a guiding light during difficult times, providing a perspective that goes beyond the present problems.

Reflect on Core Values: Identify and consider the core values that influence decisions and behaviors. Aligning problems with these values fosters a feeling of purpose and strengthens a resilient mindset.

Set Meaningful Goals: In addition to accomplishing personal goals, think about how actions affect oneself and others. Setting goals that promote a sense of meaning and purpose boosts intrinsic motivation and resilience.

Engage in Meaningful Activities: Take part in activities that correspond with your personal ideals and provide a sense of fulfillment. Meaningful activities boost resilience, whether they involve volunteering, creative endeavors, or connecting with a cause.

CHAPTER 4

The significance of quality sleep is frequently overlooked in today's fast-paced world. The importance of sleep for overall health, well-being, and longevity cannot be emphasized.

This thorough guide digs into the science of sleep, the implications of sleep deprivation, and practical tactics for improving your sleep habits, ensuring that each night is revitalizing and transforming.

The Science of Sleep

Understanding the science of sleep is essential for comprehending its importance in maintaining physical and mental health. Sleep is a complex physiological process with multiple stages, each serving a specific purpose.

Sleep stages: The sleep cycle is divided into two stages: non-rapid eye movement (NREM) and rapid eye movement (REM) sleep. NREM sleep is divided into three stages, each of which becomes deeper, whereas

REM sleep is connected with vivid dreams and cognitive restoration.

Circadian rhythms: Our internal biological clock, also known as the circadian rhythm, regulates the sleep-wake cycle. This cycle regulates the timing of sleep, hormone release, and other physiological processes, bringing them in line with the natural day-night cycle.

Hormonal Regulation: During sleep, the body produces vital hormones such as growth hormone and melatonin. Melatonin governs the sleep-wake cycle and works as a potent antioxidant, whereas growth hormone promotes physical growth and repair.

The Consequences of Sleep Deprivation

The consequences of sleep deprivation go far beyond feeling tired the next day. Chronic sleep deprivation has serious consequences for physical and mental health, impairing cognitive function, emotional well-being, and general vigor.

Sleep deprivation decreases cognitive skills like attention, memory, and decision-making. Prolonged sleep deprivation can result in decreased awareness, trouble concentrating, and an increased risk of accidents.

Sleep deprivation is strongly associated with mood problems such as anger, anxiety, and sadness. Adequate sleep is critical for emotional control and resiliency.

Sleep is essential for immune system function. Chronic sleep deprivation impairs the immune system, making people more vulnerable to infections and jeopardizing the body's ability to heal.

Metabolic Dysregulation: Lack of sleep alters hormonal homeostasis, impacting appetite-regulating hormones including leptin and ghrelin. This imbalance may lead to weight gain, insulin resistance, and an increased risk of metabolic diseases.

The Pillars of Optimal Sleep Practice

Creating a foundation for optimum sleep requires a comprehensive approach that covers a variety of lifestyle factors and sleep hygiene habits. To cultivate a healthy sleep schedule, consider the following pillars:

Consistent Sleeping Schedule: Going to bed and waking up at the same time every day, even weekends, helps maintain the body's internal clock. Consistency maintains the circadian rhythm, resulting in improved sleep quality.

Create a Sleep-Conducive Environment: Design your sleeping area to promote relaxation and comfort. This includes a comfy mattress and pillows, low noise and light levels, and a sleep-friendly room temperature.

Mindful Pre-Sleep habit: Establishing a pre-sleep habit tells the body it's time to relax. To ease the shift from wakefulness to sleep, engage in relaxing activities like reading, moderate stretching, or meditation.

Restrict Stimulants and Electronics: Caffeine and nicotine are stimulants that can disrupt sleep, so restrict your intake, especially in the hours coming up to bedtime. Furthermore, the blue light emitted by electronic devices interferes with melatonin generation, so avoid screens before bedtime.

Regular physical activity has been related to better sleep quality. Aim for at least 30 minutes of moderate exercise most days, but avoid strenuous workouts near bedtime.

Mindful Nutrition: A large dinner before bedtime might be unpleasant, but a light snack high in sleep-promoting nutrients may be beneficial. Incorporate foods rich in tryptophan, melatonin, and magnesium, such as turkey, almonds, and leafy greens, into your nighttime routine.

Sleep Hygiene (Restorative Sleep)

Sleep hygiene entails forming habits and routines that encourage restorative sleep. Implementing these methods promotes an appropriate sleep environment and improves the body's natural sleep-wake cycle.

Nighttime routines: Creating consistent nighttime routines tells the body that it's time to relax. This could involve things like reading a book, having a warm bath, or practicing relaxation techniques.

Temperature and Lighting: Keep the bedroom cool and dark to produce an optimal sleeping environment. Consider using blackout curtains, setting the thermostat at a comfortable temperature, and reducing artificial light sources.

Limit Daytime Naps: While brief naps can be rejuvenating, taking too many during the day can interfere with your nocturnal sleep. If you snooze often, aim for 20-30 minutes early in the afternoon.

Reduce your screen time at least one hour before bedtime. Phones, tablets, and computers emit blue light, which suppresses melatonin production and disrupts the natural transition to sleep.

Reserve the Bed for Sleep: Avoid using the bed for anything other than sleeping and personal relationships. This helps train the brain to identify the bed with rest, making it simpler to fall asleep when bedtime comes.

Limit Liquid Intake before Bed: While staying hydrated is important, drinking too much liquid close to bedtime might cause disturbing nightly awakenings. Try to restrict fluids in the hour or two before bedtime.

Managing Sleep Disorders

Persistent sleep difficulties may indicate a sleep condition, such as insomnia, sleep apnea, or restless legs syndrome. If sleep issues persist despite following ideal sleep practices, professional help is required.

Consulting a Sleep Specialist: Sleep specialists, such as sleep medicine physicians or licensed sleep therapists, can perform comprehensive exams to diagnose sleep disorders. They may propose additional assessments, such as sleep studies, to obtain more information.

Cognitive behavioral therapy for insomnia (CBT-I): CBT-I is a systematic therapeutic method that has been shown to effectively treat insomnia. It targets the ideas and actions that lead to sleep problems, assisting individuals in developing better sleeping patterns.

Continuous Positive Airway Pressure (CPAP) Therapy: People with sleep apnea may benefit from CPAP therapy, which involves using a machine to deliver a steady stream of air to keep their airways open while sleeping. This treatment effectively alleviates sleep apnea symptoms.

The Effect of Lifestyle on Sleep Practices.

Lifestyle decisions have a big impact on sleep practices. Certain habits and actions might help or hinder your capacity to get restorative and refreshing sleep.

Alcohol and sleep: Alcohol may cause drowsiness at first, but it disrupts the sleep cycle and prevents the transition to deeper sleep stages. Limit your alcohol consumption, particularly in the hours coming up to bedtime.

Caffeine Sensitivity: Caffeine sensitivity varies, but it's best to restrict your intake, especially in the afternoon and evening. Caffeine can be found in many unexpected places, including certain pharmaceuticals and energy beverages.

Stress Management: Chronic stress is a key cause of sleep problems. Incorporate stress management practices, such as mindfulness, deep breathing exercises, or yoga, into your everyday routine to help you relax.

Balancing Work and Rest: Maintaining appropriate sleep practices requires balancing work responsibilities with the requirement for regular rest. Prioritize sleep as an essential component of your overall well-being.

The link between sleep and lifespan is complex, with plenty of research demonstrating the tremendous impact of quality sleep on overall health and the aging process.

During deep sleep, the body goes through important cellular repair and growth processes. This involves the release of growth hormone, which is essential for tissue and organ integrity.

Adequate sleep is essential for a healthy immune system. Sleep increases the creation of immune cells and antibodies, which improves the body's ability to fight infections and illnesses.

Sleep is essential for cognitive performance, memory consolidation, and learning. During sleep, the brain analyzes and organizes information obtained during the day, which contributes to healthy mental functioning.

CHAPTER 5

Creating Personalized Medication Plans for Personal Health.

Understanding the individual's health profile, addressing unique needs, and enhancing treatment outcomes are all necessary components of creating a tailored drug plan.

Let's go into the world of tailored pharmaceutical programs, studying the function of medications and supplements in improving individual health and wellness.

Traditionally, medical treatments have been one-size-fits-all, with pharmaceuticals prescribed according to defined protocols. However, personalized medicine acknowledges individuals' inherent diversity, taking into account factors such as genetics, lifestyle, and environmental impacts.

Advances in genomic research have laid the groundwork for individualized medicine. Understanding an individual's genetic makeup enables healthcare practitioners to customize pharmaceutical regimens to genetic variances, improving efficacy and reducing potential negative effects.

Medication programs are now more precisely tailored to the unique aspects of a person's disease. Precision medicine considers the molecular and genetic characteristics of diseases, allowing drugs to target specific pathways involved in the disease process.

Medications as Precision Tools for Targeting Underlying Causes

In the area of tailored pharmaceutical programs, the emphasis switches from simply managing symptoms to addressing the root causes of health problems. Medications become precision tools, refined to address the distinct biological elements that contribute to an individual's health problems.

Individualized Therapies: Certain medical illnesses, such as cancer, necessitate individualized treatment plans. Targeted therapies, which try to interfere with specific chemicals involved in the growth and spread of cancer cells, demonstrate the precision of modern drug regimens.

Pharmacogenomics: Pharmacogenomic testing examines an individual's genetic composition to anticipate how they will react to certain drugs. This information helps healthcare providers choose treatments that are more likely to be successful and well-tolerated depending on a patient's genetic profile.

The Role of Supplements in Bridging Nutritional Gaps

Supplements, such as vitamins, minerals, and herbal remedies, complement the tailored strategy by filling nutritional gaps and improving general health.

Integrating supplements into a pharmaceutical regimen necessitates a detailed understanding of a person's eating habits, lifestyle, and special health requirements.

Supplements play an important role in treating vitamin deficits that can lead to health problems. For example, vitamin D supplements are frequently advised for those who do not get enough sun exposure, as they address inadequacies associated with bone health, immunological function, and overall well-being.

Supporting Specific Health Goals: Customizing supplement regimens to support specific health goals is an important aspect of individualized supplementing. Athletes may benefit from supplements that improve performance and recuperation, whereas people with certain dietary limitations may require supplements to address nutritional deficiencies.

Herbal Supplements and Traditional Medicine: Including herbal supplements and traditional medicine in tailored treatment programs demonstrates a comprehensive approach to health. Certain herbal medicines may help manage disorders including anxiety, sleeplessness, and digestive issues, supplementing conventional pharmaceuticals as part of a holistic regimen.

Chronic diseases frequently demand a complex approach involving drugs, lifestyle changes, and supplements. Personalized treatment strategies for chronic diseases consider the complexities of these ailments and seek to maximize long-term care.

Cardiometabolic Health: Managing illnesses such as hypertension and diabetes necessitates a tailored approach that may include a combination of drugs, dietary changes, and certain supplements. Omega-3 fatty acids, for example, have been examined for their possible cardiovascular advantages and may be included in the diet of those with heart health concerns.

Mental Health: Personalized medicine programs for mental health illnesses like depression or anxiety may include psychotropic medications, psychotherapy, and lifestyle changes. Nutritional supplements such as omega-3 fatty acids and certain vitamins may also be used to improve mental health.

Immunosuppressive drugs are frequently used to treat autoimmune illnesses, which are characterized by an excessive immune response.

Personalized treatment approaches for autoimmune disorders may include changing medication dosages based on individual responses and adding supplements to address nutritional deficiencies that are typical in these conditions.

Personalized Medication Plans for Aging Populations

As people age, their attitude to medication planning evolves to meet age-related health changes and improve general well-being. Balancing the advantages and hazards of drugs is critical in customized care for older persons.

Polypharmacy Considerations: Polypharmacy, or the use of many drugs at the same time, may be more prevalent in older persons. Personalized programs include a thorough examination of prescriptions to reduce side effects, handle potential drug interactions, and ensure that the benefits **outweigh the risks.**

Cognitive Health: Older persons' medication programs frequently include considerations for cognitive health. Omega-3 fatty acids, antioxidants, and certain vitamins may be investigated to improve brain function and lower the risk of age-related cognitive decline.

Bone Health: Addressing bone health is a common consideration in personalized programs for older people. Osteoporosis preventive medications can be taken with vitamin D and calcium supplements to improve bone density and minimize the risk of fracture.

6. Collaboration among healthcare providers and individuals

Personalized medicine plans necessitate active engagement between healthcare providers and patients. This collaborative approach relies heavily on open communication, shared decision-making, and continuing assessments of the plan's performance.

Individual Health objectives: Understanding an individual's health objectives is critical for developing a personalized approach. Whether the goal is to manage chronic illnesses, improve overall well-being, or address specific symptoms, tailoring the strategy to individual needs increases engagement and adherence.

For longevity and optimal aging, the strategic use of supplements has emerged as a key component of personalized health plans. While a well-balanced diet forms the foundation of a healthy lifestyle, supplements play a complementary role by addressing specific nutritional needs, supporting bodily functions, and potentially promoting longevity.

This book delves into the strategic use of supplements, unraveling the science behind their application and offering insights into how they can be integrated into a holistic approach for a longer and healthier life.

The Landscape of Longevity (Understanding the Aging Process)

Before delving into the strategic use of supplements, it's crucial to comprehend the complex landscape of aging. Aging is a multifaceted process influenced by genetic, environmental, and lifestyle factors. Cellular damage, inflammation, and a decline in the body's regenerative capacity contribute to the gradual deterioration of organs and tissues over time.

Cellular Senescence: Cellular senescence, the state in which cells lose their ability to divide and function, is a hallmark of aging. Accumulation of senescent cells contributes to chronic inflammation and various age-related diseases.

Oxidative Stress: Oxidative stress, resulting from an imbalance between free radicals and antioxidants in the body, is implicated in the aging process. Excessive oxidative stress can damage cellular components and accelerate aging.

Genetic and Epigenetic Factors: Genetic and epigenetic influences play a significant role in determining the rate of aging. While genetics sets the foundation, environmental factors and lifestyle choices can modulate gene expression and impact the aging trajectory.

Promoting longevity involves addressing cellular health, targeting mechanisms that influence cellular senescence, and fostering resilience against age-related damage. Certain supplements have shown promise in supporting cellular health and combating the aging process.

Nicotinamide Adenine Dinucleotide (NAD+): NAD+ is a coenzyme critical for cellular energy production and DNA repair. Levels of NAD+ decline with age, contributing to cellular dysfunction. NAD+ precursors, such as nicotinamide riboside (NR) and nicotinamide mononucleotide (NMN), have gained attention as potential supplements to boost NAD+ levels and support cellular function.

Coenzyme Q10 (CoQ10): CoQ10 is an antioxidant and a key player in the production of cellular energy (ATP). As cellular energy production tends to decline with age, supplementing with CoQ10 may support mitochondrial function and overall cellular vitality.

Mitochondrial Support: Mitochondria, the energy-producing powerhouses of cells, are central to the aging process. Supplements such as acetyl-L-carnitine, alpha-lipoic acid, and PQQ (pyrroloquinoline quinone) are believed to support mitochondrial function and may contribute to longevity by enhancing cellular energy production.

Hormonal Support for Healthy Aging

Hormonal changes are a natural part of aging, and certain supplements aim to support hormonal balance, contributing to overall well-being as individuals age.

Dehydroepiandrosterone (DHEA): DHEA is a precursor to sex hormones, and its levels decline with age. Some studies suggest that DHEA supplementation may have anti-aging effects, influencing factors such as muscle mass, bone density, and cognitive function.

Melatonin: Melatonin, known for its role in regulating sleep-wake cycles, also exhibits antioxidant properties. As melatonin production decreases with age, supplementation may support sleep quality, circadian rhythm regulation, and potentially contribute to overall health and longevity.

Adaptogens: Adaptogens are a class of herbs that may help the body adapt to stress and maintain balance. Rhodiola rosea, ashwagandha, and holy basil are examples of adaptogens that may support hormonal equilibrium and resilience to stress, contributing to healthy aging.

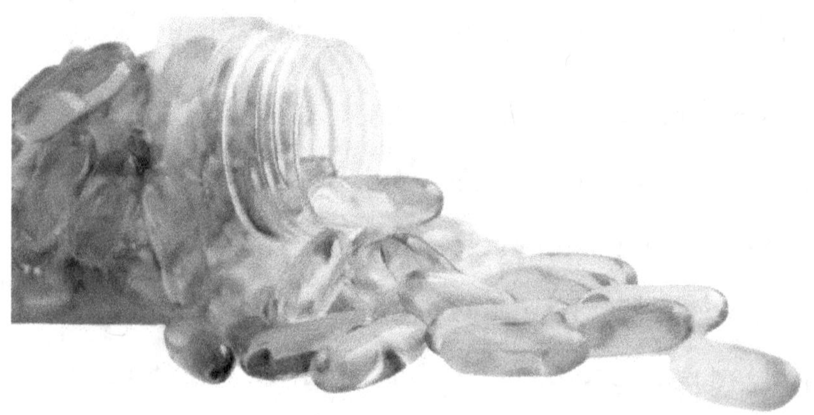

Preserving cognitive function is a key aspect of aging well. Certain supplements are believed to support brain health and may play a role in preventing or slowing down age-related cognitive decline.

Phosphatidylserine: Phosphatidylserine is a phospholipid that plays a role in maintaining cell structure and function, especially in brain cells. Supplementation may support cognitive function and memory, particularly in older adults.

Ginkgo Biloba: Ginkgo biloba is an herbal supplement that has been studied for its potential cognitive benefits. It may improve blood flow to the brain, have antioxidant effects, and support cognitive function, making it a subject of interest for brain longevity.

A robust immune system is crucial for longevity, as it defends the body against infections, reduces inflammation, and supports overall health. Several supplements are recognized for their immune-supporting properties.

Vitamin C: Vitamin C is an essential nutrient with potent antioxidant properties. It plays a crucial role in immune function by supporting the production and function of white blood cells. Supplementation with vitamin C may be considered, especially during periods of increased immune stress.

Zinc: Zinc is a trace element that is essential for immune function. It is involved in the development and function of immune cells. Adequate zinc levels support the body's ability to mount an effective immune response, and supplementation may be beneficial, particularly for individuals with deficiencies.

Probiotics: The gut microbiome plays a significant role in immune function. Probiotics, which are beneficial bacteria, support a healthy balance of gut microbiota and may enhance the body's immune response. Probiotic supplements can be considered for maintaining gut health and supporting overall immune resilience.

Considerations for Optimal Absorption and Bioavailability

The effectiveness of supplements hinges not only on their selection but also on their absorption and bioavailability. Several factors influence the body's ability to absorb and utilize nutrients from supplements.

Nutrient Synergy: Some nutrients exhibit enhanced absorption when taken together. For example, vitamin D absorption is optimized when taken with vitamin K2. Consideration of nutrient synergies enhances the strategic use of supplements for longevity.

Bioavailability: The form of a supplement influences its bioavailability, or the rate at which it is absorbed and utilized by the body. Choosing bioavailable forms of supplements ensures that the **nutrients are effectively absorbed and utilized.**

Individual Variability: Individuals may vary in their ability to absorb and utilize certain nutrients. Genetic factors, digestive health, and medication interactions can influence the individual response to supplements. Personalized approaches consider these variabilities for optimal results.

The Importance of Regular Monitoring and Adaptation

The effectiveness of a supplementation strategy is not static; it requires regular monitoring and adaptation based on changing health needs, lifestyle factors, and emerging research. Integrating regular health assessments, blood tests, and consultation with healthcare providers ensures that the supplement regimen aligns with evolving health goals.

Blood Tests and Biomarkers: Periodic blood tests can assess nutrient levels, hormonal balance, and other biomarkers relevant to aging and longevity. Adjusting supplement dosages based on these assessments allows for personalized and targeted support.

Healthcare Professional Guidance: Collaboration with healthcare professionals, including nutritionists, dietitians, and physicians, is crucial for navigating the nuanced landscape of supplementation. Their expertise helps tailor supplement plans to individual health profiles, addressing specific concerns and optimizing outcomes.

Potential Risks and Cautionary Considerations

While supplements can be powerful tools for supporting longevity, it's essential to approach their use with caution and awareness of potential risks.

Quality and Purity: The quality of supplements can vary significantly. Choosing reputable brands that adhere to quality and purity standards reduces the risk of contamination and ensures the efficacy of the supplements.

Dosage Considerations: Excessive doses of certain supplements can have adverse effects. It's important to adhere to recommended dosages and consult with healthcare professionals, especially when combining multiple supplements.

Interaction with Medications: Some supplements may interact with medications, potentially affecting their efficacy or causing adverse reactions. Individuals taking medications should consult their healthcare providers before initiating supplement regimens.

Balancing Medications with Lifestyle Options

In the complicated dance of health and wellness, the interaction of drugs and lifestyle choices is critical. While drugs are effective tools for addressing a variety of health disorders, the importance of lifestyle cannot be overemphasized.

1. Medications as a catalyst for change.

Medications are frequently accelerators for change, addressing specific health issues and alleviating symptoms. They aim to address underlying physiological mechanisms, treat chronic illnesses, and improve general well-being. However, by making attentive lifestyle choices, pharmaceutical effectiveness can be boosted and, in some cases, optimized.

Compliance and Adherence: The success of any drug regimen is dependent on patient compliance and adherence. Incorporating drugs into everyday routines, providing reminders, and appreciating the significance of consistent use all lead to better treatment outcomes.

Educational Empowerment: Knowing the purpose and potential negative effects of drugs allows people to actively engage in their health journey. Patients who are well-informed about their drugs are more likely to follow prescribed regimens and make collaborative decisions with their healthcare providers.

2. Personal Lifestyle Considerations

Recognizing the individuality of people and their lifestyles is critical to striking a harmonic balance between drugs and daily decisions. Age, gender, cultural background, and socioeconomic situation are all elements to consider while designing a personalized lifestyle.

Cultural sensitivity: Cultural variables can have a substantial impact on lifestyle choices and health habits. Healthcare providers must be culturally sensitive in their approach, recognizing the cultural background in order to make individualized advice that reflect patients' values and preferences.

Socioeconomic Impact: Economic circumstances can influence access to healthy food, physical activity opportunities, and medication adherence. A comprehensive strategy takes into account the socioeconomic situation, creating realistic and sustainable lifestyle options that respect people's budgetary limits.

Life Stage Transitions: As people progress through life stages, their lifestyle needs change. Pediatric, adolescent, adult, and geriatric groups may have different lifestyle preferences. Recognizing the specific demands of each life stage inspires specialized solutions that are responsive to individuals' changing situations.

Cognitive Effects: Medications that alter cognitive function may necessitate lifestyle changes to promote brain health. Engaging in mentally challenging activities, maintaining social connections, and prioritizing sleep all help to improve cognitive well-being.

3. Collaborative decision-making with healthcare providers.

The ability to balance drugs with lifestyle changes requires effective coordination between individuals and healthcare providers. This collaborative method entails open communication, shared decision-making, and a common understanding of the individual's health objectives.

Informed Decision-Making: Healthcare providers play an important role in educating patients about the potential effects of lifestyle choices on their health and the efficacy of medications. Individuals can actively shape their own health trajectories by making informed decisions.

Setting shared health goals helps healthcare practitioners and individuals work together more effectively. These goals include not only managing specific health issues, but also promoting overall well-being through lifestyle choices that improve medication effectiveness.

Regular Monitoring and Adjustments: Because health is a dynamic process, the factors that influence medication effectiveness may vary over time. Regular monitoring of health indicators, drug efficacy, and lifestyle adherence enables timely adjustments to improve outcomes.

4. Mind-Body Connection: Stress and Mental Health

The mind-body connection is a significant predictor of health. Stress, anxiety, and mental health all have an impact on pharmaceutical effectiveness and people's general well-being.

Stress Management Techniques: Chronic stress can alter the body's response to drugs and worsen some health disorders. Mindfulness, meditation, and deep breathing exercises are examples of stress management practices that not only improve mental health but also improve drug efficacy.

Mental Health Support: Individuals with mental health issues frequently benefit from a comprehensive strategy that includes medication, psychotherapy, social support, and lifestyle changes. The integration of these components tackles the complexities of mental health and improves overall well-being.

5. Lifestyle Choices and Chronic Disease Management.

Chronic diseases may require long-term drug regimens. Lifestyle choices become more important in the holistic management of chronic illnesses, influencing disease development, symptom management, and overall quality of life.

Cardiovascular Health: Lifestyle choices such as a heart-healthy diet, frequent exercise, and stress management are critical in treating hypertension and cardiovascular disease. These options supplement cardiovascular drugs, promoting long-term heart health.

Diabetes Management: People with diabetes benefit from a lifestyle that includes healthy eating, regular physical activity, and weight management. These lifestyle changes work in tandem with diabetes drugs, helping to maintain blood sugar levels and lower the risk of complications.

Respiratory Health: Lifestyle choices, such as quitting smoking, getting regular exercise, and taking care of the environment, are critical in controlling respiratory disorders like asthma and chronic obstructive pulmonary disease (COPD). Lifestyle changes increase the effectiveness of respiratory medicines and improve overall lung function.

6. Lifestyle prescriptions and integrative medicine.

Integrative medicine recognizes the synergistic link between traditional medical interventions and complementary therapies. Lifestyle prescriptions, which include individualized lifestyle suggestions, are consistent with integrative medicine principles and aim to improve health outcomes.

Dietary Prescriptions: Prescribe specific dietary interventions, such as a Mediterranean diet for cardiovascular health or anti-inflammatory foods for arthritis therapy, to improve pharmaceutical efficacy. These dietary suggestions are consistent with evidence-based nutritional guidelines.

Physical activity prescriptions: Exercise prescriptions that are tailored to individual fitness levels and health conditions help to improve overall well-being. Physical activity prescriptions can be combined with medication to achieve certain health goals, such as improving cardiovascular fitness, losing weight, or increasing mobility.

Mind-Body Prescriptions: Mind-body practices like yoga, tai chi, and guided relaxation provide comprehensive approaches to mental health and stress management. Integrating these activities with mental health drugs promotes a holistic approach to wellness.

CHAPTER 6

Avoiding Stupidity: Mitigating Risks for Longevity through Common-Sense Prevention

In the pursuit of longevity, it's not just about the groundbreaking strategies or cutting-edge interventions; sometimes, it's about avoiding the seemingly obvious pitfalls and adopting common-sense preventive measures.

This book explains the concept of "avoiding stupidity" in the context of longevity – identifying common risks that may undermine health and well-being and outlining practical, preventive measures to mitigate these risks.

The Not-So-Stupid Reality

Common Risks That Impact Longevity

Before delving into preventive measures, it's essential to recognize some of the everyday risks that, despite their apparent simplicity, can significantly impact longevity.

These risks are often intertwined with lifestyle choices, behaviors, and environmental factors.

Poor Dietary Choices: Despite the abundance of information on healthy eating, poor dietary choices persist as a common risk factor for various health issues. Excessive intake of processed foods, sugary beverages, and a lack of essential nutrients can contribute to obesity, cardiovascular problems, and other chronic conditions.

Sedentary Lifestyle: The modern sedentary lifestyle, characterized by prolonged periods of sitting and minimal physical activity, poses a significant risk to longevity. Physical inactivity is associated with obesity, cardiovascular diseases, and metabolic disorders.

Smoking and Tobacco Use: Tobacco use remains a major risk factor for premature death. Smoking is linked to numerous health issues, including respiratory diseases, cardiovascular problems, and an increased risk of cancer.

Excessive Alcohol Consumption: While moderate alcohol consumption may have certain health benefits, excessive drinking poses serious risks. It can lead to liver disease, cardiovascular issues, and contribute to mental health issues.

Inadequate Sleep: Sleep is a fundamental aspect of health, and chronic sleep deprivation or poor sleep quality can impact physical and mental well-being. Sleep deficiency is associated with an increased risk of obesity, diabetes, and cardiovascular diseases.

Stress and Mental Health: Chronic stress and untreated mental health conditions can have a profound impact on longevity. They are linked to an increased risk of heart disease, immune system suppression, and other health issues.

Unsafe Practices: Engaging in risky behaviors, whether in the form of reckless driving, neglecting safety precautions, or substance abuse, can lead to accidents and injuries that significantly compromise longevity.

The Wisdom of Prevention: Practical Measures for Longevity

Preventing the detrimental impact of these common risks involves adopting practical measures grounded in wisdom and common sense. The following strategies encompass a holistic approach to health, emphasizing prevention as a key component of longevity.

A. Nourishing the Body (Embrace a Nutrient-Rich Diet)

Eating a balanced and nutrient-dense diet is foundational to longevity. Focus on whole foods, including fruits, vegetables, whole grains, lean proteins, and healthy fats. Prioritize a variety of colorful fruits and vegetables to ensure a broad spectrum of vitamins, minerals, and antioxidants.

Hydration Matters: Proper hydration is often underestimated but is crucial for various bodily functions. Water supports digestion, nutrient absorption, temperature regulation, and overall cellular function. Make a conscious effort to stay adequately hydrated throughout the day.

Moderation in All Things: Adopt a balanced approach to eating by embracing the principle of moderation. While enjoying occasional treats is part of a fulfilling life, moderation helps prevent the negative consequences of excessive calorie intake, such as weight gain and metabolic disturbances.

B. Moving Towards Longevity

Incorporate Regular Exercise: Physical activity is a cornerstone of longevity. Aim for at least 150 minutes of moderate-intensity aerobic exercise or 75 minutes of vigorous-intensity exercise per week, along with muscle-strengthening activities on two or more days a week. Find activities you enjoy to make exercise a sustainable part of your routine.

Break Up Sedentary Time: Combat the hazards of prolonged sitting by incorporating regular breaks and movement throughout the day. Stand up, stretch, or take short walks, especially if your job involves long periods of sitting. Simple movements can have a profound impact on overall health.

Strength Training for Resilience: Include strength training exercises in your routine to enhance muscle strength, bone density, and overall resilience. Resistance training, whether through weights, resistance bands, or bodyweight exercises, contributes to a strong and functional body.

Mind-Body Practices: Consider integrating mind-body practices such as yoga or tai chi into your routine. These practices not only enhance physical flexibility and balance but also promote mental well-being, stress reduction, and a sense of calm.

C. Abandoning Harmful Habits

Quit Smoking: If you smoke, quitting is one of the most impactful decisions for your longevity. Smoking cessation significantly reduces the risk of heart disease, respiratory issues, and various cancers. Seek support from healthcare professionals or smoking cessation programs to increase your chances of success.

Moderate Alcohol Consumption: If you consume alcohol, do so in moderation. The definition of moderate drinking varies, but it generally means up to one drink per day for women and up to two drinks per day for men. Excessive alcohol consumption has well-documented health risks, including liver disease and cardiovascular problems.

Create a Sleep Sanctuary: Prioritize sleep as a non-negotiable aspect of your daily routine. Create a sleep-conducive environment by keeping the bedroom dark, quiet, and cool. Establish consistent sleep patterns, aiming for 7-9 hours of quality sleep per night. Adequate and restful sleep supports physical and mental well-being.

D. Managing Stress and Nurturing Mental Health

Stress Management Techniques: Develop effective stress management techniques to mitigate the impact of chronic stress on your health. Techniques such as deep breathing, meditation, mindfulness, and progressive muscle relaxation can help reduce stress levels and promote relaxation.

Prioritize Mental Health: Mental health is an integral component of longevity. Seek professional help if you're experiencing persistent feelings of anxiety, depression, or other mental health issues. Addressing mental health challenges is a proactive step towards overall well-being.

Cultivate Social Connections: Social connections play a vital role in mental and emotional well-being. Nurture relationships with friends, family, and community. Engage in activities that foster a sense of belonging and connection, as social support is a powerful protective factor against the negative impact of stress.

E. Safety First: Practical Measures for Accident Prevention

Practice Safe Driving: Adopt safe driving practices to reduce the risk of accidents. Avoid distracted driving, obey traffic laws, and use seat belts consistently. Defensive driving techniques contribute to personal safety and longevity.

Home Safety Measures: Make your home environment safe by addressing potential hazards. Install smoke detectors, use non-slip mats in bathrooms, secure handrails on staircases, and ensure adequate lighting. These simple measures can prevent accidents and injuries, particularly in older age.

Avoiding Substance Abuse: Steer clear of substance abuse, including recreational drugs. Substance abuse not only poses immediate risks but can also contribute to chronic health issues and mental health disorders. Seeking support for substance abuse concerns is a crucial step towards a healthier and longer life.

Lifelong Learning: The Intellectual Fountain of Youth

Cognitive Stimulation: Engage in activities that stimulate cognitive function and promote brain health. Reading, solving puzzles, learning new skills, and pursuing lifelong learning opportunities keep the brain active and resilient against age-related cognitive decline.

Embrace Curiosity: Cultivate a mindset of curiosity and openness to new experiences. Embracing novelty, whether through travel, hobbies, or intellectual pursuits, fosters a sense of purpose and contributes to mental and emotional well-being.

Social Intellectual Engagement: Participate in intellectually stimulating conversations and activities within your social circles. Engaging with others in discussions, debates, or collaborative projects provides mental stimulation and contributes to a rich and fulfilling life.

Preventive Health Screenings (Proactive Healthcare for Longevity)

Regular Health Check-ups: Schedule regular health check-ups and screenings as recommended by healthcare professionals. Early detection and management of health issues contribute to better outcomes and can prevent the progression of certain conditions.

Know Your Numbers: Be aware of key health indicators such as blood pressure, cholesterol levels, and blood sugar levels. Understanding these numbers empowers you to make informed decisions about lifestyle and, if necessary, to collaborate with healthcare providers on intervention strategies.

Vaccinations: Stay up-to-date with vaccinations to protect against preventable diseases. Vaccinations are a crucial aspect of preventive healthcare and contribute to overall immunity, reducing the risk of infections that can impact longevity.

Environmental Awareness

Environmental Stewardship: Contribute to environmental well-being by adopting sustainable practices. Environmental factors, including air and water quality, can impact health. Supporting initiatives that promote clean environments benefits both personal health and the well-being of future generations.

Sun Safety: Practice sun safety to protect against harmful UV radiation. Use sunscreen, wear protective clothing, and seek shade, especially during peak sun hours. Protecting the skin from sun damage reduces the risk of skin cancer and premature aging.

Clean and Safe Living Spaces: Ensure that your living spaces are clean and safe. Address environmental hazards such as mold, pollutants, and other potential health risks. A healthy living environment supports overall well-being and contributes to longevity.

A Wise Path to Longevity

Avoiding stupidity in the pursuit of longevity involves adopting a wise and practical approach to health. While groundbreaking advancements in medical science and innovative interventions are valuable, the foundation of longevity lies in everyday choices and preventive measures. Nourishing the body with wholesome nutrition, embracing physical activity, quitting harmful habits, managing stress, prioritizing mental health, ensuring safety, engaging in lifelong learning, proactive healthcare, and environmental awareness collectively form a holistic strategy for a longer and healthier life.

The journey to longevity is not about perfection but about making informed choices that align with the principles of well-being. It's a journey guided by the wisdom of prevention, where individuals take charge of their health, cultivate resilience, and foster a life that not only spans the years but is filled with vitality, purpose, and fulfillment.

As we navigate the complexities of modern life, let us embrace the simplicity of avoiding stupidity and walk the path to longevity with mindful steps and a heart filled with the wisdom of well-lived days.

Avoiding Stupidity

The pursuit of health is not only about adopting positive practices but also about avoiding unnecessary dangers and pitfalls. This book explains the concept of "Avoiding Stupidity" with a focus on practical strategies for mitigating risks that could jeopardize well-being and compromise the journey towards a longer and healthier life.

1. Understanding the Nature of Unnecessary Dangers

Unnecessary dangers, often rooted in impulsive decisions, lack of awareness, or neglect, can significantly impact health and longevity. These dangers may manifest in various aspects of life, including lifestyle choices, safety practices, and mental well-being. Identifying these potential risks is the first step in crafting strategies to avoid them.

Reckless Lifestyle Choices: Unhealthy habits, such as poor dietary choices, sedentary behavior, and substance abuse, contribute to avoidable health risks. Addressing these lifestyle choices is crucial for preventing long-term health issues.

Neglecting Safety Precautions: Ignoring safety precautions, whether at home, on the road, or in recreational activities, can lead to accidents and injuries. Neglecting safety measures increases the likelihood of avoidable harm.

Overlooking Mental Well-being: Mental health is an integral component of longevity. Neglecting mental well-being, ignoring signs of stress or mental health conditions, can have profound consequences on overall health and quality of life.

2. Developing a Mindful Approach to Daily Choices

Avoiding unnecessary dangers begins with cultivating mindfulness in daily choices. Mindfulness involves being fully present, aware, and intentional in each moment. By incorporating mindfulness into decision-making processes, individuals can steer clear of impulsive or reckless actions that may compromise their well-being.

Conscious Physical Activity:

Mindful physical activity means engaging in exercises with awareness and intention. Whether it's a brisk walk, yoga, or weightlifting, being present in the moment enhances the benefits of physical activity while minimizing the risk of injury.

Safety Precautions in Daily Life

From using seat belts in the car to wearing safety gear during recreational activities, incorporating safety precautions into daily life is a conscious choice. These measures reduce the likelihood of accidents and injuries.

Emotional Awareness and Stress Management:

Emotional awareness involves recognizing and understanding one's emotions. By being emotionally aware, individuals can address stressors proactively and implement effective stress management techniques to prevent the negative impact of chronic stress on health.

Many unnecessary dangers arise from the pursuit of instant gratification without considering the long-term consequences. Prioritizing health and well-being over momentary pleasures requires a shift in mindset and a commitment to long-term goals.

Choosing Nutrient-Rich Foods:

Opting for nutrient-rich foods over processed and indulgent choices is a conscious decision for long-term health. While the latter may provide immediate satisfaction, the former supports overall well-being and longevity.

Regular Exercise for Sustainable Health:

Engaging in regular exercise might not yield immediate results, but its cumulative benefits contribute to sustained health and vitality. Prioritizing consistent physical activity is a key strategy for avoiding the unnecessary dangers of a sedentary lifestyle.

Responsible Substance Use:

Whether it's alcohol, tobacco, or recreational drugs, adopting a responsible approach to substance use involves considering the long-term impact on health. Balancing moderation and awareness mitigates the risks associated with substance abuse.

Creating a Safe and Supportive Environment

Avoiding unnecessary dangers extends beyond personal choices to the environment in which individuals live and work. Creating a safe and supportive environment involves implementing measures that reduce potential risks and enhance overall well-being.

Home Safety Measures:

Conducting a home safety assessment and implementing necessary measures, such as installing smoke detectors, securing handrails, and ensuring proper lighting, reduces the risk of accidents and injuries within the home.

Workplace Safety Practices:

Employers and employees alike play a role in maintaining a safe workplace. Adhering to safety protocols, using protective equipment, and promoting a culture of safety contribute to a work environment that minimizes unnecessary dangers.

Cultivating Supportive Relationships:

Surrounding oneself with supportive and positive relationships is a protective factor for mental well-being. Strong social connections act as a buffer against stress and contribute to a sense of security and belonging.

Learning from Mistakes and Adjusting Course

Avoiding stupidity involves acknowledging that mistakes can happen but using them as opportunities for growth and learning. Instead of dwelling on errors, individuals can adopt a resilient mindset, learn from their experiences, and adjust their course to make better-informed decisions in the future.

Reflecting on Past Choices:

Regular self-reflection on past choices, both positive and negative, enhances self-awareness. Acknowledging mistakes without self-judgment allows individuals to identify patterns, understand triggers, and make informed adjustments.

Embracing a Growth Mindset:

Embracing a growth mindset involves viewing challenges and setbacks as opportunities for learning and improvement. Rather than seeing mistakes as failures, individuals with a growth mindset recognize them as stepping stones on the path to personal development.

Seeking Professional Guidance:

In situations where decisions have significant consequences, seeking professional guidance is a wise strategy. Whether it's consulting with a healthcare professional, a safety expert, or a mental health professional, expert advice can provide valuable insights for making informed choices.

Mental well-being is a cornerstone of avoiding unnecessary dangers. Integrating mental health strategies into daily life is essential for resilience, stress management, and overall longevity.

Mindfulness and Meditation:

Incorporating mindfulness and meditation practices into daily routines enhances mental clarity, reduces stress, and fosters a calm and focused mindset. Regular practice strengthens emotional resilience and supports overall well-being.

Therapeutic Techniques:

Therapeutic techniques, such as cognitive-behavioral therapy (CBT) or dialectical behavior therapy (DBT), provide tools for managing emotions, improving decision-making, and navigating challenging situations. Seeking therapeutic support is a proactive step towards mental well-being.

Open Communication:

Open communication with trusted friends, family, or mental health professionals creates a supportive network. Sharing thoughts and feelings reduces the burden of emotional stress and fosters a sense of connection and understanding.

Cultivating Adaptability in the Face of Change

Life is dynamic, and unforeseen circumstances are inevitable. Cultivating adaptability is a powerful strategy for navigating changes, minimizing risks, and promoting longevity.

Flexibility in Decision-Making:

Being flexible in decision-making involves adapting to new information and adjusting plans accordingly. Rigidity can lead to unnecessary dangers, while flexibility allows for a more adaptive and responsive approach to life's challenges.

Embracing Life Transitions:

Life transitions, whether related to career, relationships, or health, require adaptability. Embracing change with a positive mindset and seeking support when needed promotes resilience and contributes to overall well-being.

Learning New Skills:

Actively pursuing opportunities to learn new skills enhances adaptability. Acquiring new knowledge and abilities equips individuals to face diverse challenges and navigate different aspects of life with confidence.

Maintaining a Holistic Perspective on Longevity

Avoiding unnecessary dangers for longevity involves adopting a holistic perspective that considers the interconnectedness of physical, mental, and emotional well-being. A comprehensive approach recognizes that health is multifaceted and requires attention to various aspects of life.

Holistic Healthcare Practices:

Integrating holistic healthcare practices, including complementary and alternative therapies, into one's routine supports overall well-being. Practices such as acupuncture, massage, or herbal medicine can complement conventional medical approaches.

Balancing Work and Life:

Striking a balance between work and personal life is crucial for avoiding burnout and sustaining longevity. Implementing boundaries, prioritizing self-care, and fostering a healthy work-life balance contribute to overall well-being.

Connection with Nature:

Spending time in nature has been linked to numerous health benefits, including stress reduction, improved mood, and enhanced cognitive function. Whether through outdoor activities, gardening, or simply taking a walk in the park, connecting with nature supports longevity.

Avoiding stupidity in the pursuit of longevity is about making thoughtful choices, being aware of potential dangers, and prioritizing well-being over immediate gratification.

By incorporating mindfulness into daily decisions, prioritizing health, creating a safe environment, learning from mistakes, integrating mental health strategies, cultivating adaptability, and maintaining a holistic perspective, individuals can navigate the complexities of life with wisdom and resilience.

The journey to a longer life is not about avoiding all risks but about making informed choices that contribute to overall well-being. It's a path guided by thoughtful strategies, where individuals actively engage with the present moment, learn from experiences, and cultivate a life that is not only longer but also filled with purpose, fulfillment, and meaningful connections. In the tapestry of longevity, the threads of mindful living weave a resilient and vibrant narrative, ensuring that each step is taken with conscious intent and a heart set on the horizon of a healthy and fulfilling future

1. Nourishing the Body: The Nutrient-Rich Foundation

A nutrient-rich diet is the cornerstone of the longevity lifestyle. The foods we consume provide the building blocks for every aspect of our physical well-being. The personalized playbook emphasizes the following principles for nourishing the body:

Whole Foods and Diversity: Prioritize whole, minimally processed foods, embracing a diverse array of fruits, vegetables, whole grains, lean proteins, and healthy fats. The rich tapestry of nutrients in a varied diet supports overall health.

Hydration as a Habit: Staying adequately hydrated is often underestimated but is crucial for optimal bodily functions. Cultivate the habit of regular hydration, recognizing the role water plays in digestion, nutrient absorption, and cellular processes.

Balanced Nutrition for Every Stage: Recognize the evolving nutritional needs at different life stages. From childhood to adolescence, adulthood, and beyond, tailor nutritional choices to support the body's changing requirements.

2. Moving with Purpose: Physical Activity as a Lifelong Companion

Physical activity is not just a component of the longevity lifestyle; it's a lifelong companion that contributes to vitality and well-being. The personalized playbook emphasizes the following principles for incorporating physical activity:

Consistency over Intensity: Consistency in physical activity often outweighs intensity. Establish a routine that is sustainable over the long term, incorporating activities you enjoy. Regular, moderate exercise has cumulative benefits for health and longevity.

Mind-Body Integration: Recognize the mind-body connection in physical activity. Practices like yoga, tai chi, or mindful walking not only contribute to physical fitness but also enhance mental well-being, stress management, and overall resilience.

Lifelong Movement: Embrace the concept of lifelong movement. Physical activity is not confined to a particular age; it evolves with you. Stay active throughout the different life stages, adapting your routine to accommodate changing needs and preferences.

3. Cultivating Mental Resilience: The Mindset Matters Approach

The longevity lifestyle places a strong emphasis on mental resilience and a positive mindset. Cultivating mental well-being is integral to overall health. The personalized playbook underscores the following principles for fostering mental resilience:

Positive Self-Talk: Be mindful of your inner dialogue. Positive self-talk contributes to a resilient mindset and enhances your ability to navigate challenges. Replace self-limiting beliefs with affirmations that empower and uplift.

Adaptability and Growth Mindset: Embrace adaptability and a growth mindset. Life is dynamic, and challenges are inevitable. Viewing setbacks as opportunities for learning and growth fosters resilience and a proactive approach to life.

Stress Management Techniques: Develop a repertoire of stress management techniques. Whether it's mindfulness meditation, deep breathing exercises, or engaging in hobbies that bring joy, these practices contribute to emotional well-being and longevity.

Identify and cultivate meaning and purpose in your life. Having a sense of direction and contributing to something larger than yourself enhances mental resilience and provides a framework for making meaningful choices.

4. Prioritizing Quality Sleep: The Restorative Pillar

Sleep is a non-negotiable pillar of the longevity lifestyle. The personalized playbook highlights the significance of quality sleep for physical and mental well-being:

Sleep Hygiene Practices: Establish consistent sleep hygiene practices to create a conducive sleep environment. This includes keeping the bedroom dark, cool, and quiet, and minimizing screen time before bedtime. Quality sleep sets the stage for optimal health.

Regular Sleep Patterns: Aim for regular sleep patterns by going to bed and waking up at consistent times. Aligning your sleep schedule with your natural circadian rhythm supports the body's internal clock and enhances the restorative quality of sleep.

Mindful Wind-Down Routine: Develop a mindful wind-down routine before bedtime. Engage in relaxing activities, such as reading, gentle stretching, or practicing gratitude. Creating a transition from the busyness of the day to a restful night promotes sleep quality.

Addressing Sleep Disorders: If sleep issues persist, seek professional guidance to address potential sleep disorders. Identifying and treating conditions such as sleep apnea or insomnia is essential for maintaining overall health and longevity.

5. Harmonizing Lifestyle Components:

The longevity lifestyle is not a collection of isolated practices but an interconnected web where each component influences the others. The personalized playbook emphasizes the harmonization of lifestyle components:

Balanced Integration: Integrate dietary choices, physical activity, mental resilience practices, and sleep into a balanced and cohesive lifestyle. Recognize that the synergy between these elements amplifies their individual benefits.

Holistic Health Screenings: Prioritize regular health check-ups and screenings to proactively monitor your health. Early detection and intervention contribute to the holistic approach of preventive healthcare.

Mindful Decision-Making: Approach lifestyle choices with mindfulness and intention. Whether it's choosing a meal, deciding on an exercise routine, or managing stress, mindful decision-making aligns actions with long-term health goals.

Adapting to Life Transitions: Life is marked by transitions, and the longevity lifestyle accommodates these changes. Whether it's a career shift, family dynamics, or age-related adjustments, adapting with resilience and a focus on well-being is paramount.

6. Personalized Nutrition:

The concept of personalized nutrition is integral to the longevity lifestyle. Recognizing that individuals have unique nutritional needs, the personalized playbook emphasizes the following principles:

Bioindividuality: Acknowledge your bioindividuality – the idea that each person has unique nutritional requirements based on factors such as genetics, metabolism, and lifestyle. Tailor your nutrition choices to suit your individual profile.

Functional Foods: Integrate functional foods into your diet – foods that provide health benefits beyond basic nutrition. Examples include berries with antioxidants, fatty fish with omega-3 fatty acids, and cruciferous vegetables with anti-inflammatory properties.

Nutrigenomics: Explore the field of nutrigenomics, which examines how individual genetic variations influence responses to specific nutrients. Understanding your genetic predispositions can guide personalized dietary choices for optimal health.

7. Avoiding Stupidity: Mitigating Risks for Longevity

Avoiding unnecessary dangers is a key principle of the longevity lifestyle. The personalized playbook emphasizes strategies for mitigating risks and making thoughtful choices:

Conscious Decision-Making: Approach decisions with consciousness and intention. Whether it's dietary choices, physical activities, or safety measures, conscious decision-making minimizes the risk of avoidable dangers.

Learning from Mistakes: Acknowledge that mistakes may happen, but view them as opportunities for learning and growth. Reflect on past choices, adjust course when needed, and cultivate a mindset of continuous improvement.

Safety First: Prioritize safety in various aspects of life, from driving practices to home safety measures. Creating a safe and supportive environment reduces the likelihood of accidents and contributes to overall well-being.

8. Environmental Awareness

The longevity lifestyle extends its focus beyond personal choices to environmental awareness. The personalized playbook emphasizes the following principles:

Environmental Stewardship: Contribute to environmental well-being by adopting sustainable practices. Supporting initiatives that promote clean environments benefits both personal health and the well-being of future generations.

Sun Safety Practices: Practice sun safety to protect against harmful UV radiation. Use sunscreen, wear protective clothing, and seek shade, especially during peak sun hours. Protecting the skin from sun damage reduces the risk of skin cancer and premature aging.

Clean and Safe Living Spaces: Ensure that your living spaces are clean and safe. Address environmental hazards such as mold, pollutants, and other potential health risks. A healthy living environment supports overall well-being and contributes to longevity.

9. Unified Lifestyle Plan:

The longevity lifestyle isn't a rigid set of rules but a unified lifestyle plan that harmoniously integrates the principles outlined in the personalized playbook. The personalized playbook emphasizes:

Synergy of Components: Recognize the interconnectedness of various lifestyle components. The synergy between nutrition, physical activity, mental resilience, sleep, and other aspects amplifies the overall benefits, promoting holistic well-being.

Adaptability and Flexibility: Embrace adaptability and flexibility in your lifestyle plan. Life is dynamic, and the ability to adjust your approach based on changing circumstances ensures that your longevity lifestyle remains sustainable and fulfilling.

Individualized Strategies: Tailor the longevity lifestyle to your unique preferences, needs, and goals. The personalized playbook provides a framework, but individualized strategies ensure that the lifestyle plan aligns with your specific profile and fosters a sense of ownership.

CHAPTER 7

Blue Zone Wisdom: Lessons from the World's Longest-Lived Cultures

These longevity hotspots offer profound insights into the lifestyle, habits, and mindset that contribute to a long and healthy life. As we delve into the Blue Zone wisdom, we uncover the key principles that can inspire and guide us on our own journey towards a more vibrant and extended life.

1. Centenarians as Role Models

In the Blue Zones, reaching the age of 100 is not a rarity but a norm. These regions, including places like Okinawa (Japan), Sardinia (Italy), Nicoya Peninsula (Costa Rica), Ikaria (Greece), and Loma Linda (California, USA), are home to a significant number of centenarians. One of the first lessons from the Blue Zones is the value of these individuals as role models.

Centenarians in Blue Zones often share common lifestyle traits such as an active daily routine, strong social connections, and a diet rich in plant-based foods. Learning from their experiences and adopting some of these lifestyle elements can provide valuable insights into the choices that contribute to a long and healthy life.

2. Plant-Based Nutrition:

A consistent theme across Blue Zones is the emphasis on plant-based nutrition. The majority of the diet in these regions consists of vegetables, fruits, whole grains, legumes, and nuts. Plant-based diets are not only rich in essential nutrients but also contribute to lower rates of chronic diseases.

In Okinawa, for instance, the traditional diet is characterized by the consumption of sweet potatoes, tofu, and a variety of vegetables. Similarly, in Ikaria, the Mediterranean diet with an abundance of olive oil, vegetables, and herbs is a staple.

The emphasis on plant-centric meals in Blue Zones highlights the importance of choosing nutrient-dense, whole foods for optimal health and longevity.

3. Social Connectivity

Blue Zones underscore the significance of strong social connections in promoting longevity. The communities in these regions prioritize family bonds, close-knit social networks, and regular interactions. These connections provide emotional support, a sense of belonging, and contribute to reduced stress levels.

In Okinawa, for example, the concept of "moai" represents a social support group that starts in childhood and lasts throughout life. The power of community is evident in the longevity of Okinawans. Similarly, in Nicoya, Costa Rica, the "plan de vida," or life plan, is shaped by strong social bonds and a sense of purpose within the community.

Embracing the Blue Zone wisdom of fostering meaningful connections in our own lives can positively impact not only our mental and emotional well-being but also our overall life expectancy.

4. Purposeful Living:

Blue Zone residents often lead lives filled with purpose and meaning. The concept of "ikigai" in Okinawa, which translates to "a reason for being," emphasizes the importance of having a sense of purpose. Whether it's through meaningful work, contributing to the community, or nurturing familial relationships, the people in Blue Zones find purpose in their daily lives.

This emphasis on purposeful living aligns with research suggesting that having a strong sense of purpose is associated with better mental health, resilience, and longevity. Incorporating elements of "ikigai" into our own lives can involve exploring our passions, engaging in activities that bring joy, and cultivating a sense of purpose that extends beyond age.

5. Daily Physical Activity: Moving Naturally

Unlike modern sedentary lifestyles, Blue Zone communities engage in daily physical activities that are integrated into their lives. Whether it's walking, gardening, or performing household chores, the residents of Blue Zones move naturally throughout the day. This constant, low-intensity physical activity contributes to their overall health and longevity.

In Ikaria, for instance, the hilly terrain encourages regular walking, while in Sardinia, the practice of walking to neighbors' houses, tending to livestock, and working in the fields keeps individuals active. Embracing the wisdom of incorporating natural movement into our daily routines can be a simple yet effective way to enhance our well-being.

6. Stress Reduction Practices:

Stress reduction is an integral part of the Blue Zone lifestyle. Residents engage in practices that promote relaxation and mental well-being. Whether it's through daily rituals, mindfulness practices, or a strong sense of community support, stress reduction is woven into the fabric of daily life.

In Ikaria, the afternoon "siesta" is not just a nap but a time to unwind and relax. Similarly, in Okinawa, the practice of "nagomi" encourages forgiveness and the release of grudges, contributing to reduced stress levels. Adopting stress reduction practices from Blue Zones, such as mindfulness meditation or spending time in nature, can positively impact our mental health and contribute to overall longevity.

7. Moderate Alcohol Consumption:

Moderate and regular alcohol consumption is a common thread in several Blue Zones. In Sardinia, for instance, the consumption of red wine is a part of daily life. The key here is moderation, with an emphasis on the social aspect of sharing a drink with friends or family.

The antioxidants present in red wine are believed to have potential health benefits. However, it's crucial to note that excessive alcohol consumption can have detrimental effects on health. Embracing the Blue Zone wisdom of moderate and mindful alcohol consumption underscores the importance of balance in lifestyle choices.

8. Connection with Nature:

Blue Zone communities often have a close connection with nature. Whether it's the coastal beauty of Ikaria, the green hills of Sardinia, or the lush landscapes of Costa Rica, the residents are surrounded by natural environments. This connection with nature contributes to lower stress levels, enhanced mental well-being, and a more active lifestyle.

Research suggests that spending time in nature is associated with various health benefits, including improved mood, reduced stress, and enhanced cognitive function. Incorporating nature into our daily lives, whether through outdoor activities, gardening, or simply taking a stroll in a nearby park, aligns with the Blue Zone wisdom of nurturing well-being through a connection with the natural world.

9. Family-Centric Values:

In Blue Zones, family plays a central role in the lives of residents. Multi-generational households are common, and there's a strong tradition of care and support across generations. This familial support not only contributes to the well-being of individuals but also provides a sense of security and belonging.

In Nicoya, for instance, the elderly are often actively involved in childcare, contributing to a sense of purpose and connection. Embracing family-centric values and cultivating close relationships with family members can be a source of emotional support and well-being, aligning with the Blue Zone wisdom of prioritizing family bonds.

10. Blue Zone Environment:

The physical environment of Blue Zones itself plays a role in promoting longevity. The natural landscapes, clean air, and community-oriented design contribute to a supportive ecosystem for well-being. This environment encourages healthy lifestyle choices, outdoor activities, and a sense of community.

While not everyone can live in a designated Blue Zone, adopting elements of their environment, such as creating green spaces in urban areas, promoting walkable neighborhoods, and fostering a sense of community, can positively impact our own well-being.

The Blue Zone wisdom provides a treasure trove of insights that can inspire us to lead healthier, more fulfilling lives. While we may not replicate every aspect of life in a Blue Zone, integrating key principles into our daily routines can contribute to enhanced well-being and longevity.

Whether it's adopting a more plant-based diet, prioritizing social connections, finding purpose in daily activities, or embracing stress reduction practices, the lessons from Blue Zones offer practical and achievable steps. The journey towards a longer and healthier life is not about perfection but about making intentional choices that align with the core principles of well-being found in these longevity hotspots.

As we navigate the complexities of modern life, the Blue Zone wisdom serves as a beacon, reminding us of the timeless principles that contribute to a life well-lived. By incorporating these lessons into our own lifestyles, we can embark on a journey towards longevity, embracing not only the quantity but the quality of the years ahead.

The Blue Zone wisdom becomes a guide, urging us to savor each moment, cultivate meaningful connections, and nurture a sense of purpose that transcends age – a timeless blueprint for a vibrant and enduring life.

Women's Health

Women's health is a multifaceted and dynamic journey that encompasses physical, mental, and social well-being. From adolescence to menopause and beyond, women navigate unique challenges and experiences that shape their overall health. This comprehensive exploration explains the various aspects of women's health, addressing key considerations, preventive measures, and empowering practices that contribute to a thriving and fulfilling life.

1. The Foundation:

Women's health is a holistic concept that extends beyond reproductive concerns to encompass the entire spectrum of well-being. While reproductive health is a crucial component, a comprehensive approach recognizes the interconnection between physical, mental, and social dimensions. Holistic health empowers women to prioritize self-care, cultivate positive habits, and make informed choices that resonate with their unique needs.

Understanding women's health holistically involves acknowledging the influence of biological, psychological, and social factors. From hormonal fluctuations to societal expectations, women navigate a complex interplay of influences that impact their health at different life stages. Recognizing this complexity forms the foundation for fostering well-being across the lifespan.

2. Adolescence:

The transition from girlhood to womanhood during adolescence is a critical phase that sets the stage for lifelong health. Physical and emotional changes, onset of menstruation, and the development of body image contribute to the unique challenges faced by adolescent girls.

3. Nutrition and Physical Activity:

Adequate nutrition is essential during adolescence to support growth and development. Encouraging a balanced diet rich in nutrients, along with regular physical activity, lays the foundation for a healthy lifestyle. It also contributes to bone health, which is particularly crucial during this stage.

Menstrual Health Education: Comprehensive menstrual health education is imperative to empower adolescent girls with knowledge about their bodies. Understanding menstrual cycles, proper hygiene practices, and addressing menstrual stigma are key components of promoting reproductive health during adolescence.

Mental Health Support: Adolescence is a time of heightened emotional sensitivity. Providing mental health support, fostering self-esteem, and addressing body image concerns contribute to overall well-being. Open communication channels between parents, educators, and healthcare providers are crucial in creating a supportive environment.

3. Reproductive Years:

The reproductive years mark a significant period in women's lives, characterized by menstrual cycles, fertility considerations, and the potential for pregnancy. Nurturing reproductive health involves addressing menstrual health, family planning, and supporting women during pregnancy and childbirth.

Menstrual Health and Hygiene: Menstrual health extends beyond adolescence, requiring ongoing attention throughout the reproductive years. Promoting menstrual hygiene, addressing menstrual pain, and understanding menstrual irregularities contribute to overall well-being.

Family Planning and Fertility Awareness:

Women's health during the reproductive years often involves family planning decisions. Access to comprehensive family planning resources, fertility awareness, and discussions about reproductive choices empower women to make informed decisions aligned with their life goals.

Pregnancy and Postpartum Care: Pregnancy is a transformative journey that necessitates specialized care. Access to prenatal care, nutritional support, and emotional well-being during pregnancy contribute to maternal health. Postpartum care, including mental health support and resources for new mothers, is equally vital.

4. Menopause:

Menopause represents a natural life transition for women, signaling the end of reproductive years. While it brings hormonal changes and potential challenges, menopause is not a medical condition but a normal part of aging. Approaching menopause with a positive mindset and adopting healthy practices can significantly impact women's well-being during this phase.

Hormonal Changes and Symptom Management: Hormonal fluctuations during menopause can lead to symptoms such as hot flashes, mood changes, and sleep disturbances. While these are common, their impact varies among women. Management strategies may include lifestyle modifications, hormonal therapies, or alternative approaches based on individual preferences and health considerations.

Bone Health and Cardiovascular Health: Menopause is associated with a decline in estrogen levels, impacting bone health and cardiovascular health. Prioritizing calcium and vitamin D intake, engaging in weight-bearing exercises, and adopting heart-healthy habits contribute to overall health during and after menopause.

Mental Health and Emotional Well-Being: Menopause can influence mental health, with some women experiencing mood changes or an increased risk of depression. Open communication about these changes, seeking support, and addressing mental health concerns contribute to a positive menopausal experience.

5. Mental Health:

Mental health is an integral component of women's overall well-being. Women may face unique mental health challenges, influenced by biological, psychological, and sociocultural factors. Breaking stigmas surrounding mental health, fostering resilience, and promoting supportive environments are crucial for women at every life stage.

Common Mental Health Concerns: Women may be more prone to conditions such as depression and anxiety, influenced by hormonal fluctuations, life transitions, and societal pressures. Recognizing the signs of mental health concerns and seeking timely support are essential for effective management.

Stress Management: Balancing multiple roles and responsibilities, women often experience high levels of stress. Incorporating stress management techniques such as mindfulness, relaxation exercises, and time management strategies supports mental well-being.

Postpartum Depression and Perinatal Mental Health: The postpartum period is a vulnerable time for mental health. Awareness, routine screening, and accessible mental health resources are essential components of perinatal mental health care.

6. Preventive Health Measures:

Empowering women with knowledge about preventive health measures is a cornerstone of promoting overall well-being. Regular health check-ups, screenings, and lifestyle modifications contribute to early detection and effective management of potential health risks.

Regular Health Check-Ups: Routine health check-ups are vital for preventive care. Regular screenings for breast health, cervical health, and other relevant examinations contribute to early detection and timely interventions.

Breast Health Awareness: Breast health awareness, including self-examinations and regular mammograms as recommended, is crucial for the early detection of breast conditions. Educational initiatives and accessible screening programs contribute to women's health.

Heart Health Awareness: Cardiovascular health is a significant consideration for women. Awareness of heart disease risk factors, lifestyle modifications such as healthy eating and regular exercise, and routine cardiovascular screenings contribute to heart health.

7. Healthy Lifestyle Practices:

Adopting healthy lifestyle practices forms the bedrock of women's health. From nutrition and physical activity to sleep hygiene and stress management, lifestyle choices profoundly influence overall well-being.

Balanced Nutrition: A balanced and nutrient-rich diet is fundamental for women's health. Emphasizing whole foods, incorporating a variety of fruits and vegetables, and maintaining adequate hydration contribute to optimal nutrition.

Regular Physical Activity: Physical activity is crucial for maintaining a healthy weight, supporting cardiovascular health, and promoting overall well-being. Engaging in regular exercise, including both aerobic and strength-training activities, is recommended.

Adequate Sleep: Quality sleep is essential for physical and mental restoration. Establishing a consistent sleep routine, creating a conducive sleep environment, and addressing sleep disorders contribute to restorative sleep.

Stress Reduction Techniques: Stress reduction techniques, including mindfulness, meditation, and relaxation exercises, are invaluable for mental well-being. Integrating these practices into daily life supports stress management.

8. Empowering Women through Education and Access

Empowering women with education and access to healthcare resources is fundamental to fostering well-being. From reproductive health education to access to family planning services, comprehensive healthcare empowers women to make informed choices about their bodies and lives.

Reproductive Health Education: Comprehensive reproductive health education equips women with knowledge about their bodies, menstrual health, family planning options, and sexual health. Accessible information contributes to informed decision-making.

Family Planning Services: Access to family planning services, including contraceptives and reproductive health consultations, is essential for women to make choices aligned with their life goals. These services contribute to maternal health and overall well-being.

Maternal Health Services: Adequate maternal health services, including prenatal care, childbirth support, and postpartum care, are crucial for the well-being of both mothers and infants. Access to these services contributes to positive pregnancy and childbirth experiences.

9. Social Support and Community Engagement

Social support and community engagement play pivotal roles in women's health. Building strong social connections, fostering supportive communities, and addressing social determinants of health contribute to overall well-being.

Community Resources: Access to community resources, including women's health clinics, support groups, and educational initiatives, enhances overall health. Community engagement fosters a sense of belonging and connection.

Work-Life Balance: Balancing work and personal life is a common challenge for women. Advocating for work-life balance, flexible work arrangements, and supportive workplace policies contribute to both professional success and personal well-being.

Addressing Social Determinants of Health: Recognizing and addressing social determinants of health, such as socioeconomic factors, education, and housing, is crucial for achieving health equity. Initiatives that address these determinants contribute to improved health outcomes for women.

10. Menstrual Equity and Advocacy

Menstrual equity involves ensuring that all women have access to menstrual products, education, and support without facing stigma or barriers. Addressing menstrual equity contributes to women's dignity, health, and participation in various aspects of life.

Access to Menstrual Products: Ensuring affordable and accessible menstrual products is essential for menstrual hygiene. Initiatives that provide free or subsidized products contribute to menstrual equity.

Education and Destigmatization: Comprehensive menstrual health education destigmatizes menstruation and promotes open conversations. Advocacy for menstrual equity involves challenging taboos and ensuring that menstruation is recognized as a natural and normal bodily function.

Empowering Women for a Lifetime of Well-Being

Women's health is a dynamic journey that encompasses various life stages, challenges, and triumphs. Fostering well-being involves a holistic approach that addresses physical, mental, and social dimensions. From adolescence to menopause and beyond, empowering women with knowledge, access to healthcare, and supportive communities contributes to a lifetime of well-being.

By recognizing the uniqueness of women's health needs, embracing preventive measures, and advocating for health equity, we create a foundation for healthier generations.

The journey towards women's well-being is a shared responsibility that involves individuals, communities, healthcare providers, and policymakers working collaboratively to empower women to lead fulfilling lives at every stage. As we celebrate the achievements and resilience of women, let us also commit to nurturing a world where every woman has the opportunity to thrive, flourish, and achieve her highest potential across the lifespan.

CONCLUSION

In the vibrant artwork of human existence, the thread of health weaves intricate patterns that influence every part of our journey. As we traverse the maze of life, our bodies bear witness to the decisions we make, repeating the consequences of our acts and inactions.

The narrative of our health develops in the pages of our daily lives, a story rife with possibility yet riddled with problems. In our quest for longevity and vitality, we have arrived at a fork in the road, where the path to well-being beckons with promise and possibilities.

The quest to health is a never-ending voyage, a sacred agreement between mind, body, and spirit. It's a symphony of balance, a dance between sustenance and activity, rest and regeneration, resilience and renewal. However, in the cacophony of modern life, surrounded by deadlines and diversions, it is all too easy to overlook the very vessel that takes us through the waves of time.

The revelation in this book is a beacon of light, revealing the path to robust living and immortal energy. Within its pages are the keys to unlocking the mysteries of well-being, providing a road map for overcoming the constraints of age and disability. We find the alchemy of transformation by combining mindful nutrition, energizing exercise, restorative sleep, and the elixir of hydration.

However, the ultimate definition of health goes beyond the absence of illness; it is a condition of wholeness, a balance of body, mind, and spirit. The glow of joy illuminates our eyes, the power propels us ahead, and the tranquility anchors us in the face of life's storms. It is the richness that is greater than all treasures, the money of life itself.

As guardians of our own well-being, we are charged with a sacred duty: to honor and cherish the vessel of our life, and to tend to its requirements with reverence and care. For the sanctuary of our bodies contains the essence of our humanity, the reservoir of our dreams and aspirations, and the temple of our soul.

Let us heed the wisdom revealed within these pages, treating each nugget of insight as a priceless jewel, a treasure trove of knowledge to help us on our journey to completeness. Let us build a culture of self-care in which every bite, every movement, and every breath is imbued with intention and attention.

May we be stewards of our own health, protecting the flame of vitality that burns inside. May we regain our entitlement to radiant living, and accept each passing year as proof of the human spirit's resiliency. And may we inspire others to start on this transformative journey, instilling hope in hearts tired from the responsibilities of life.

For, in the end, it is not the years in our lives that matter, but the lives we lead. Let us grab each moment with zeal, relishing the symphony of feelings, the kaleidoscope of experiences that constitute our common humanity. And may the wisdom in this book serve as a guiding star, illuminating the route to a fulfilling life and leaving a legacy of health and happiness for future generations.

Daily Journal

Daily Journal

Daily Journal

Daily Journal

Daily Journal

Daily Journal

Daily Journal

Daily Journal

Daily Journal

Daily Journal